The Health Plan for Overweight Children

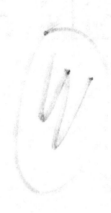

The Health Plan for Overweight Children

A Parent's Guide to Raising a Healthier Child

Dr. Melissa Langone

iUniverse, Inc.
New York Lincoln Shanghai

The Health Plan for Overweight Children
A Parent's Guide to Raising a Healthier Child

iUniverse books may be ordered through booksellers or by contacting:

iUniverse
2021 Pine Lake Road, Suite 100
Lincoln, NE 68512
www.iuniverse.com
1-800-Authors (1-800-288-4677)

Because of the dynamic nature of the Internet, any Web addresses or links contained in this book may have changed since publication and may no longer be valid.

ISBN: 978-0-595-44939-2 (pbk)
ISBN: 978-0-595-69099-2 (cloth)
ISBN: 978-0-595-89261-7 (ebk)

Printed in the United States of America

This book is dedicated to my mother and father, Denise and Tom Langone. Thank you for your unwavering support, advice, and guidance.

Contents

Preface

As a health care provider, I have seen an increase in the number of children who fall into the category of being overweight or obese. As an educator, I know that with proper instruction and guidance, parents are willing to take the necessary steps to ensure the better health of their children. Often in the health care setting, health care providers do not have the time to sit down with parents and really explain the changes that are necessary in their child's diet. Having been educated both in pediatrics and in nutrition, I understand what methods work best when trying to change eating and activity patterns among children.

The Health Plan for Overweight Children involves a change in lifestyle that will benefit your child for the rest of his or her life. By following the guidelines in this book, not only will the health of your child improve, but you will also benefit from a healthier lifestyle. Every child is different, and no two children will progress with the suggested changes in this book at the same pace. By being able to individualize the rate at which you make changes to your child's eating and activity patterns, you increase your child's opportunity to be successful in following the plan.

I understand that many parents want to help their child lead a healthier lifestyle; they just lack the proper information and tools to implement these lifestyle changes. That is why I wrote the Health Plan for Overweight Children, to provide parents with the tools they need to begin creating a healthier lifestyle for their child. The ultimate goal of this plan is to create a society of children with healthier hearts, bodies, and minds.

CHAPTER 1

INTRODUCTION

This book is designed to provide you with the information needed to make your child as healthy as possible. If you have an overweight child, you are not alone. The number of children who fall into the category of being overweight or obese continues to increase. The effects of being overweight as a child can last long into adulthood and make the risk of heart disease, stroke, high blood pressure, and diabetes increase as your child ages.

The focus of this book is not on weight loss, it is on making your child healthier. The first and most important step you can take for your overweight child is to change your goal from: "I want my child to lose weight;" to "I want my child to be healthy." By following this plan, your child will lose weight, but this should not be the primary concern. Shifting focus from your child's weight to their health will benefit them both physically and emotionally.

This plan will be much more effective for your child if you also follow the guidelines of this book. Even though your child won't admit it until they are in their 20s or 30s (maybe), you are your child's role model. What you do and say affects not only what your child does but also how they feel about themselves. If your child sees you leading an unhealthy lifestyle, they are going to resist any change to their eating and activity patterns.

Some parents have turned to the use of medications and surgery to help their child lose weight. Weight loss medications can have many side effects and some can even cause dependency. The long-term effects of many of these medications are unknown. Some people believe that surgery is the best option for their child. After surgery that is performed to make the stomach smaller, a person can only consume approximately 800 calories per day. For a growing child, this type of caloric restriction may be dangerous and can lead to vitamin deficiencies. The long-term effects of these surgeries on children are also unknown. Medications and surgery often do not deal with the emotional issues that underlie eating patterns.

You can improve the health of your child without the use of medications or surgery. The Health Plan for Overweight Children focuses on including healthy foods as part of your child's diet and activity as part of their daily routine. This plan is designed for children who are six and older because children who are younger then six have different nutritional needs. The earlier in your child's life that you begin these guidelines, the easier it will be to get your child to change their eating patterns. But, it is never too late to teach your child to make healthier choices for themselves. It may take more time and changes may be gradual for an older child, but think about the difference you will make in your child's future.

What Causes Overweight?

When people eat more food than the stomach can handle, it will make them feel uncomfortable at first. However, if they continue to eat larger portions, the stomach will stretch to accommodate for the extra volume. When the stomach is stretched, it takes more food to make someone feel full and satisfied, leading to overeating and weight gain.

The stomach can shrink back to its original size, but portion sizes must be smaller. Gradual changes in portion sizes are less likely to cause the feeling of hunger than a dramatic change. You can begin by replacing the foods your child currently consumes with healthier choices to start improving their health. When they become accustomed to the healthier foods, you can begin slowly decreasing the portion sizes to reach the amount they should be consuming for their age. Exact portion sizes that are needed depend upon the age of your child, and will be discussed in Chapter 3.

Our bodies obtain energy when we consume fats, carbohydrates, and proteins. Energy is stored in the body as glycogen, but when those stores are full, excess glycogen is converted to fat and stored. Fat cells in the body have a certain amount of fat that they can store. When that amount of fat reaches its maximum, fat cells divide. While fat cells can be made smaller, once they have divided there will always be a higher number of fat cells. Fat cells do not die or disappear they only shrink. The reason why this is dangerous is that it is easier to regain weight when you have a higher number of fat cells. Fat cells divide the most during childhood, which makes preventing or correcting obesity in childhood very important to your child's future health. Changes in your child's diet and activity patterns can affect both current and future disease risks. Unlike diet plans, the Health Plan for Overweight Children promotes changes in the diet that will help shrink fat cells by focusing on healthy foods and activity and not dwelling on weight.

In adulthood, overweight and obesity can lead to many conditions that will negatively affect health. Type II diabetes is more common in individuals who are overweight. While this type of diabetes is known as adult onset diabetes, it is becoming more and more common among children due to obesity. Cardiovascular disease and stroke are more common among overweight adults. When obesity begins at a younger age, negative effects on the cardiovascular system will happen sooner. Obesity can also cause problems with the joints because of the excessive weight that is placed on them.

I am not giving you this information to scare you, but to emphasize the importance of preventing or correcting overweight and obesity in your child. Like any parent, you want what is best for your child. By implementing the plan that is outlined in this book, you will take an important step in ensuring good health for your child now and as they continue to grow.

Summary Points

* ❖ *Focus on making your child healthy, not their weight.*
* ❖ *What you do and say effects what your child does and how they feel about themselves.*
* ❖ *The long-term effects of weight-loss surgeries and medications are unknown.*
* ❖ *Include healthy foods and regular physical activity.*
* ❖ *Include gradual changes in portion sizes.*
* ❖ *Replace current foods with healthier choices.*
* ❖ *Fat cells divide most during childhood, making the prevention or decrease in childhood obesity very important.*
* ❖ *Obesity increases the risk of type II diabetes, cardiovascular disease, and joint problems with age.*

CHAPTER 2

THE NEVER DIET AGAIN HEALTH PLAN

The Health Plan for Overweight Children is not a diet. What do you think about when you hear the word diet? Do the words temporary, deprived, or starved come to mind? Probably. Even though the word "diet" really refers to the foods that we eat, most of us think of cutting back on food when we hear the word. The Health Plan for Overweight Children is a lifestyle. It's about changing how you and your child think about food and concentrating on becoming healthy.

At no point in this book will I tell you to eliminate a food or category of foods from your child's diet. I may suggest limiting a food, but never eliminating a food. Even cake, cookies, soda, and fast food will not be eliminated, just limited. What happens when someone tells you that you can't have a food? Most of the time, it makes you want that food more. Children should be allowed to have birthday cake, drink soda at a party, or occasionally go to a fast food restaurant with friends. It only becomes a problem when children make these choices on a regular basis.

Carbohydrates are not an evil food as some have tried to make it seem. They are extremely important to your child's diet. Even fat is essential for a growing child, but there are different types of fat. I will teach you how to choose the right fats for your child. If you follow this health plan, your child will never feel deprived of food or starved.

Say Goodbye to the Scale

If you do not own a scale, *do not* go out and buy one. If you do own a scale, put it away. Again, the focus of this plan is not on weight loss, it is on health. Even body mass index (BMI), which compares your child's weight to their height, can be inaccurate. The BMI does not consider body composition. For example, if you have a child who is very muscular, it is possible that your child will fall into an overweight BMI category even though they have a healthy body. If you are weighing your child on a daily or weekly basis, they know that weight is your primary concern. You may be telling your child with words that you want them to be healthy, but by weighing your child, your actions are telling them that you want them to lose weight. Save the weighing of your children for when they visit their pediatrician or health care provider.

Dangers of a Weight Focused Plan

Focusing on weight can lead to low self-esteem in your child, and I will discuss this more in the Emotional Eating chapter. Another problem with focusing on weight is the potential to contribute to eating disorders. While being overweight is unhealthy for your child, being underweight is just as unhealthy.

Anorexia Nervosa is an eating disorder that develops when people starve themselves to lose weight. When the body is deprived of nutrients, the body turns to its own stores to provide them. The body will begin breaking down muscle, including the heart, to provide energy to the body. While some children may do this to lose weight, others have a psychological condition where they cannot see themselves as they really are when they look in the mirror. Even though they are thin, they see themselves as obese.

* *Warning signs of anorexia: If your child will not eat in front of family members, skips meals or always makes excuses for missing meals, or takes very small portions of food it may be a sign of this condition. Please see your child's health care provider if your child shows these signs.*

Another eating disorder is Bulimia Nervosa, where people eat large amounts of food and then cause themselves to vomit. Many people think that in order for a person to have an eating disorder they have to be a stick thin figure. But, with bulimia, someone can be overweight and still have the condition. If someone eats more food than he or she vomits, their weight can stay at an increased level. There are many dangers of this condition. When someone is vomiting all the time they are losing elements in their body that regulate important functions like the beating of the heart. When these elements are out of balance, a heart attack may result. The acid from the stomach can also wear away the lining of the esophagus and the enamel on the teeth.

Warning signs of bulimia: If your child goes to the bathroom after every meal, if you are missing large quantities of food in a short period of time, or if the enamel on the back of your child's teeth is worn away it may be a sign of this condition. Please see your child's health care provider if your child shows these signs.

Encourage Results

When people are learning new behaviors, like eating or activity behaviors, using positive reinforcement allows the learning of new behaviors to be more successful. Rather than punishing your child or using negative comments when they do not follow the plan, praise and reward them when they do follow the plan. You can create a reward calendar like the one below. For a young child, when they exercise, choose a healthy food over an unhealthy food, or make a positive comment about themselves, you can give them a star or have them color in a star on the chart. For older kids, you can give them paper money that you have created and printed on your computer or have drawn on a piece of paper.

When your child receives a certain amount of stars or "dollars," they can receive some type of reward. It should *not* be a food reward. A toy, game, or something similar can be the reward, as long as the reward is not food. Ideally it should be a reward that will help to increase your child's physical activity, a basketball, baseball mitt, volleyball net, kite, or Frisbee are just some ideas. It is important for your child to feel like they are reaching goals, so you should use a smaller reward for a row of stars or a certain amount of "dollars" and a larger reward for a completed star sheet or collecting a larger amount of "dollars."

Health Plan Rewards									
Reward Goal: _____									
Number of Stars Needed: _____									
☆	☆	☆	☆	☆	☆	☆	☆	☆	☆
☆	☆	☆	☆	☆	☆	☆	☆	☆	☆
☆	☆	☆	☆	☆	☆	☆	☆	☆	☆
☆	☆	☆	☆	☆	☆	☆	☆	☆	☆
☆	☆	☆	☆	☆	☆	☆	☆	☆	☆
☆	☆	☆	☆	☆	☆	☆	☆	☆	☆
☆	☆	☆	☆	☆	☆	☆	☆	☆	☆

Have Fun

The Health Plan for Overweight Children will be successful if you HAVE FUN. Include:

Healthy Foods

Activity

Vitamins and Minerals

End Emotional Eating

Family Support

U as a role Model

No Focus on Weight

Including healthy foods, physical activity, and vitamins and minerals are essential to the development of a healthy child. For the psychological health of your child, finding alternatives to emotional eating will help your child cope with stress. Having support from all family members and having you as a role model will increase your child's success with this health plan. I will also teach you how to read a food label and choose better carbohydrates, fats, and proteins for your child. I will also address issues with regard to eating at school.

Summary Points

- ❖ *The Health Plan for Overweight Children is a lifestyle, not a diet.*
- ❖ *I may suggest that a food be limited, but there will be no elimination of any one food or category of foods.*
- ❖ *Carbohydrates are an extremely important part of your child's food intake.*
- ❖ *Do not weigh your child; let your child's health care provider keep track of weight.*
- ❖ *Pay attention to signs of anorexia nervosa and bulimia nervosa.*
- ❖ *Positive reinforcement aids in adopting new behaviors.*
- ❖ *Have fun, include:*
  - o *Healthy foods*
  - o *Activity*
  - o *Vitamins and minerals*
  - o *End emotional eating*
  - o *Family support*
  - o *U as a role model*
  - o *No focus on weight*

CHAPTER 3

HEALTHY FOOD SCHOOL

A healthy diet includes carbohydrates (grains, vegetables, and fruit), fats, and proteins (milk, meat, and beans). All of these foods provide the body with nutrients so that it can grow, develop, and function correctly. It is important to include foods from all of these categories into a child's daily diet and not to eliminate any categories. Based on the USDA food guide, the following are specific recommendations for your child.

Age and Gender	Grains	Vegetables	Fruit	Milk	Meat and Beans
6 year old Female	5 ounces	1.5 cups	1.5 cups	2 cups	4 ounces
6-8 year old Male 7-9 year old Female	5 ounces	2 cups	1.5 cups	3 cups	5 ounces
9-10 year old Male 10-11 year old Female	6 ounces	2.5 cups	1.5 cups	3 cups	5 ounces
11 year old Male 12-18 year old Female	6 ounces	2.5 cups	2 cups	3 cups	5.5 ounces
12-13 year old Male	7 ounces	3 cups	2 cups	3 cups	6 ounces

Age and Gender	Grains	Vegetables	Fruit	Milk	Meat and Beans
14 year old Male	8 ounces	3 cups	2 cups	3 cups	6.5 ounces
15 year old Male	9 ounces	3.5 cups	2 cups	3 cups	6.5 ounces
16-18 year old Male	10 ounces	3.5 cups	2.5 cups	3 cups	7 ounces

* Source: United States Department of Agriculture. My Pyramid. www.mypyramid.gov
Based on a child who exercises 30-60 minutes most days of the week.

Carbohydrate Class

Carbohydrates are important because they provide energy to the brain, blood cells, and nervous system. You have probably heard of simple and complex carbohydrates before. You can find simple carbohydrates in products that are easily broken down in the body and quickly raise blood sugar levels. Products that contain a lot of sugar, such as candy bars, cookies, and soda are simple carbohydrates. Complex carbohydrates take a while for your body to break down, so they do not cause that sudden increase in blood sugar. Starches are one type of complex carbohydrate, and you can find starches in cereal, grain, and bread products. Fibers are another type of complex carbohydrate, and you can find fiber in all foods that come from plants including fruits, vegetables, and grains.

Whole grain or whole-wheat products are better for your child than refined white products because they contain many nutrients of the original grain. The refining process of white bread and pasta removes many of these nutrients, including iron, zinc, and fiber. If your child does not like one brand of whole wheat bread or pasta, try a different brand. Not all whole wheat breads or pastas have the same consistency. Another option is multigrain products, which are being made more often now. There are multigrain pastas and breads that have not been through the refining process of white breads so they still have original nutrients, but they also taste similar and have a similar consistency to those products. After your child becomes used to eating multigrain foods, you can then introduce whole-wheat products to your child's diet.

Whole-wheat flour is excellent for cooking. You can substitute whole-wheat flour for white flour in breads, cakes, and pancakes. Brown rice provides many nutrients for your child. You can make a dinner combination of brown rice, vegetables, and chicken to provide your child with foods from three of the major food groups.

Depending upon the age of your child, the requirement of grain products may range from 5 ounces to 10 ounces. It is easier to meet these requirements than you might think. If your child had 1 cup of cereal for breakfast, a sandwich on whole-wheat bread for lunch, and 1 cup of rice or pasta with their dinner, it would equal 5 servings of grains. For older children, they typically eat more than one serving at a meal, which increases their intake to the necessary amounts of grains. Each product on the list below is equal to one ounce of grains:

- ❖ 1 slice of bread
- ❖ 1 cup of cereal
- ❖ ½ cup of rice
- ❖ ½ cup cooked cereal
- ❖ ½ cup pasta
- ❖ 1 mini bagel (a large bagel is equal to 4 ounces)
- ❖ 1 small biscuit
- ❖ 5 whole wheat crackers or 7 saltine crackers
- ❖ ½ English muffin
- ❖ 1 pancake
- ❖ 1 small flour or corn tortilla

* Source: United States Department of Agriculture. My Pyramid. www.mypyramid.gov

Veggie and Fruit Facts

Fruits and vegetables are carbohydrates because they are made of fiber. There have been new findings that there are nutrients called phytonutrients that are important to good health, and you can find these phytonutrients in plant products. Taking a vitamin supplement will not provide your child with these phytonutrients; you can only find them in fresh fruits and vegetables. Phytonutrients help protect the body against cell damage, protect against heart disease, and boost the immune system. Carotenoids, flavonoids, phenolic acid, and lignans act as antioxidants in the body, protecting the cells against damage. Ellagic acid, indoles, isothiocyanates, saponins, and terpenes help protect the body from cancer and tumor growth. Protease inhibitors and capsaicin help to lower inflammation in the body from conditions like arthritis (which can develop in some children). Following is a list of the phytonutrients and in what foods they can be found.

Phytonutrient	Source
Carotenoids	Red, orange, yellow, and green fruits and vegetables
Flavonoids	Almost all fruits and vegetables
Ellagic Acid	Strawberries, grapes, raspberries, and apples
Phenolic Acid	Almost all fruits and vegetables and whole grains
Indoles	Cabbage, broccoli, Brussels sprouts, kale and kohlrabi
Isothiocyanates	Cabbage, broccoli, Brussels sprouts, kale and kohlrabi
Lignans	Berries, flax seeds, and whole grains
Saponins	Garlic, onion, beans, and soybeans
Protease Inhibitors	All plants
Terpenes	Citrus Fruits
Capsaicin	Hot Peppers

Source: Beling, Stephanie. (1997) *Power Foods*. HarperCollins Publishers: New York.

The required intake of vegetables for your child ranges from 1.5 cups to 3.5 cups and for fruit, it ranges from 1.5 to 2.5 cups. The following items are equal to a one cup serving of vegetables:
   ❖ 1 cup of raw or cooked vegetables
   ❖ 1 cup of vegetable juice
   ❖ 2 cups of raw leafy green vegetables
   ❖ 1 medium boiled or baked potato

❖ 1 large baked sweet potato

A one-cup serving of fruit is equal to:

❖ 1 cup of fruit juice (100% juice only)
❖ 1 medium sized fruit or ½ large sized fruit
❖ 1 cup of chopped fruit or grapes
❖ ½ cup of dried fruit
❖ 1 cup of applesauce
❖ 8 large strawberries
❖ 1 small (1" thick) piece of watermelon

* Source: United States Department of Agriculture. My Pyramid. www.mypyramid.gov

Many people believe that it costs more to buy fresh fruits and vegetables than it does to go out and purchase food at a fast food restaurant. In chapter 4, I will show you that it is more expensive for a family of four to eat out at a fast food restaurant for all of their meals than it is to purchase fresh foods and cook your meals at home. The cost of fresh fruits and vegetables may start to add up if you purchase the foods and then do not eat them before they go bad. To prevent this, you can make meal plans for a week to make sure you do not buy more fruits and vegetables than you need. Another option is to buy bagged frozen fruits and vegetables. If you purchase produce this way, it holds on to most, if not all, of the original nutrients. You can remove the amount of fruit or vegetables that will be eaten and freeze the rest.

Canned fruit that is packaged in water is a good option for your child. Avoid canned fruits that are packaged in heavy syrup. You can add fresh fruit, like bananas or berries, to your child's cereal in the morning to increase sweetness and increase the amount of fruit they are consuming. For an easy and delicious way to encourage your child to eat fruit, try making a fruit smoothie. Use skim milk, fat free frozen yogurt and add banana, mango, papaya, or berries and mix in a blender. Your child will get the benefit of eating the whole fruit, but many times children do not consider this as eating fruit because they are drinking it and because it tastes so good. While 100% fruit juice is considered a serving of fruit, your child will not get the benefit of the fiber unless the juice has pulp. Eating whole fruits or adding whole fruits to a smoothie are great ways for your child to get the nutrients and fiber that they need.

The number of servings of fruits and vegetables, 1.5-3.5 for vegetables and 1.5-2.5 for fruit, are the minimum amounts your child should be eating every-day. But, do not place a limit on the amount of fruits and vegetables that your child can eat. Because fruits and vegetables contain fiber, they make your child feel full which helps regulate their intake. If your child wants to eat a snack, choosing a fruit or vegetable will be better than something that provides empty calories. Empty calories come from foods that will give your child energy, but little if any nutrients. Foods that provide empty calories include soda, candy, cookies, cakes, and other junk foods. By eating fruits and vegetables for snacks, your child will receive the nutrients they need.

Examples of Good Carbohydrates		
GRAINS	FRUITS	VEGETABLES
Barley Bran Brown Rice Bulgur Couscous Multigrain bread and pasta Oatmeal Whole-wheat bread/rolls Whole-wheat cereals Whole-wheat crackers Whole-wheat flower Whole-wheat pasta Whole rye Wild Rice	Apples Nectarines Apricots Oranges Bananas Papaya Berries (All) Peaches Cherries Pears Grapefruit Pineapple Grapes Plums Kiwi Tangerines Lemons Limes Mangos Melons (All) (And All Fruits Not Listed)	Artichoke Kale Asparagus Lettuce Beets Pumpkin Broccoli Parsnip Brussels sprouts Potatoes Cabbage Squash Carrots Turnip Cauliflower Celery Cucumber Eggplant Green beans Green Peppers (And All Vegetables Not Listed)

The Dish on Meat, Poultry, and Fish

Protein is important in the body because it helps to build muscle and tissues, helps to heal wounds, helps maintain a balance of fluids in the body, and allows the immune system to function. Proteins are made up of small structures called amino acids. Both plant and animal foods contain protein, but animal foods are called complete proteins because they contain all the amino acids the body requires. Plant food sources are considered incomplete because they do not contain all of the amino acids.

Most children eat much more protein from meat than they need. The number of ounces required ranges from 4 ounces to 7 ounces depending upon the age of your child. One small lean hamburger is equal to 2 to 3 ounces of meat. Lean cuts of beef and pork are better for your child than meat that is labeled as prime or choice. Prime and choice meats tend to be high in the type of fat that should be limited in your child's diet. Use lean ground beef for making hamburgers or other foods requiring chop meat. You may also want to try turkey burgers cooked with a little steak sauce to make them taste more like beef. There are also lower fat alternatives to hot dogs. The following is equal to a one ounce serving of meat:

- ❖ 1 ounce of meat, fish, or poultry
- ❖ 1 egg
- ❖ ¼ cup of cooked beans
- ❖ 2 tablespoons of hummus
- ❖ 1 tablespoon of peanut butter
- ❖ ½ ounce of nuts or seeds
- ❖ ¼ cup of tofu

* Source: United States Department of Agriculture. My Pyramid. www.mypyramid.gov

When you are purchasing poultry, like chicken and turkey, buying skinless cuts are better for your child's health. Baking or broiling meats rather than frying them will decrease the fat content. Many processed lunchmeats are high in sodium and other additives. You should avoid bologna and salami because they have the highest fat content. Choosing lower fat processed meats, like turkey and ham, will be healthier for your child.

* *Caution: Make sure you thoroughly cook meat products, keep them refrigerated until they are ready to be cooked, avoid touching uncooked meat with other foods, and wash your hands, counters, and utensils thoroughly after touching raw meat to prevent contamination with bacteria.*

Fish is a great source of protein for your child and provides your child with fats that are important to good health called Omega-3 fatty acids. Omega-3 fatty acids are important to the health of the heart, immune system, and nervous system. You can also find Omega-3 fatty acids in tofu and soybeans.

* *Caution: Certain types of fish have been found to be high in mercury, including shark, swordfish, king mackerel, and tilefish. Children and pregnant women should avoid these types of fish because they can have negative effects on your child's nervous system.*

Egg Education

Eggs are an excellent source of protein in your child's diet. Many people still associate eggs with being a bad food because they contain cholesterol. They do contain cholesterol, but not as much as was originally believed. When you consume cholesterol from food, it does not immediately become cholesterol in your blood. In fact, eating a diet high in saturated fat is more likely to raise blood cholesterol levels than dietary cholesterol. Blood cholesterol becomes dangerous when it deposits along the walls of the arteries in the body.

As long as your child does not eat them excessively, eggs can contribute to the good health of your child. Eggs contain vitamins and minerals that are important to the growth of your child and they are low in sodium. Your child should consume no more than two eggs per day. Eating more than two eggs per day will prevent your child from eating other foods that are necessary to meet their needs.

Legume Lab

Beans, which are also known as legumes, are excellent sources of fiber, iron, and calcium. Soy and other legumes help to promote the health of the heart and the building of healthy bones. Tofu is made from soybeans and can be used as a protein source for your child. Soy nuts and soymilk are another way to incorporate soy products into your child's diet.

Types of Legumes			
Baked beans	Garbanzo beans	Navy Beans	Split peas
Black beans	Kidney beans	Pinto Beans	White Beans
Black-eye peas	Lentils	Refried Beans	
Cowpeas	Lima Beans	Soy Beans	

Get Good Marks with Milk

Dairy includes cheese, yogurt, milk, and other milk products. Milk products are a great source of calcium and vitamin D, which is very important to your child's growing bones. If you usually use whole milk, you should switch to lower fat milk for your child. Whole milk contains saturated fat, the type of fat that should be limited in your child's diet. Most kids will not go directly from whole milk to skim milk. You can slowly decrease the amount of fat that is present in your child's milk. You can first use 2% milk for a few weeks, then down to 1%, and finally skim milk. Rather than ice cream, try giving your child low fat or fat-free frozen yogurt. Most kids cannot tell the difference between ice cream and frozen yogurt. A one-cup serving of milk is equal to:

❖ 1 cup of milk or yogurt

- ❖ 1 ½ ounces of natural cheese
- ❖ 2 ounces of processed cheese
- ❖ ½ cup evaporated milk
- ❖ $1/3$ cup of shredded cheese
- ❖ ½ cup ricotta cheese
- ❖ 2 cups cottage cheese
- ❖ 1 cup pudding
- ❖ 1 cup frozen yogurt
- ❖ 1 ½ cups of ice cream

* Source: United States Department of Agriculture. My Pyramid. www.mypyramid.gov

Read about Nuts and Seeds

Nuts and seeds are a great source of vitamins and minerals. Seeds include pumpkin, sesame, and sunflower seeds. Nuts include pine nuts, almonds, walnuts, hazelnuts, Brazil nuts, cashews, macadamias, pecans, and pistachios. Raw nuts are a much better choice than roasted nuts, which have higher calorie and fat content. Unsalted nuts are also a better choice because nuts that have been roasted and salted can be very high in sodium. If your child does not like unsalted nuts, try mixing them with dried fruit or adding chopped nuts to cereal in the morning. While nuts do contain fat, it is the type of fat that is good for your child. Nuts also contain the phytonutrients that were discussed under fruits and vegetables earlier in this chapter.

Cooking Class

Oil is something that most people use for cooking, but there are many different types of oil and some are better than others are. Oils are a good source of vitamin E in the diet, but those with a low amount of saturated and trans fats should be used. Polyunsaturated and monounsaturated oils are the best choices including safflower, sunflower, corn, soybean, olive, and canola oils. You should avoid oils such as coconut or palm oil and shortenings or lard. You should use other fats, like butter, with moderation in your child's diet. Margarines that contain trans fats should be avoided because of their ability to raise cholesterol levels.

Summary Points

❖ *Foods from all of the food groups should be included in your child's diet.*

❖ *Carbohydrates are an important source of energy for the brain, blood cells, and nervous system.*

❖ *Complex carbohydrates include starches and fibers.*

❖ *Whole grain and whole-wheat products are better choices than refined products.*

❖ *The daily requirement for grain products ranges from 5 to 10 ounces depending upon age and gender.*

❖ *Fruits and vegetables contain important phytonutrients.*

❖ *The daily requirement for vegetables ranges from 1.5 to 3.5 cups and for fruit ranges from 1.5 to 2.5 cups depending upon age and gender.*

❖ *Use fruits and vegetables as snacks rather than foods with empty calories.*

❖ *Protein is needed for many functions in the body.*

❖ *Purchase low fat meats and skinless poultry.*

❖ *Include fish as part of your child's diet.*

❖ *Eggs are good source of protein.*

❖ *Legumes (or beans) are a healthy addition to your child's diet.*

❖ *Low fat or nonfat dairy products are best.*

❖ *Nuts and seeds are a great source of vitamins and minerals.*

❖ *Polyunsaturated and monounsaturated oils are the best choices (safflower, sunflower, corn, soybean, olive, and canola oils).*

CHAPTER 4

FOOD FOR THE BODY AND MIND

With a little effort, eating healthy can become a way of life for your child and your family. The benefits of making better food choices include a healthier body and a healthier mind. Variety and moderation are two key words you need to learn to make your child healthy. Variety means varying the foods your child eats from day to day. Even if you find a healthy meal plan for your child, and he or she ate that meal plan every day, they would end up deficient in something. Most people eat the same thing for breakfast every day. As long as your child is eating a healthy breakfast, this is not a problem. But, lunch, dinner, and snacks should be varied every week to ensure your child receives all the nutrients needed for good health. Moderation means not eating any type of food excessively. If your child is eating one food group excessively and eliminating others, again, they can become deficient in necessary nutrients. For example, oranges are great for you. But, if you ate oranges all day, everyday, you would be missing other nutrients that are just as important to your health as the ones you are receiving from the orange.

The Deal with Meals

Our bodies use glucose for energy. The body stores glucose in the muscles and in the liver. Because children have smaller livers than adults, they do not have as much room to store extra glucose. Because of that, it is important for children to eat at least 3 meals to maintain their blood sugar levels. Small frequent meals consumed about 4-5 times per day are even more effective in maintaining those levels. While it may be possible for your child to eat small frequent meals on weekends, it is difficult to eat this way with the structure of school days. So, for most days of the week, your child should eat 3 healthy meals per day.

Feed the Brain

The most important way to start your child's day is to make sure they eat breakfast. Breakfast provides your child with energy their body desperately needs at the beginning of the day. Studies have found that children who consume breakfast have better nutrient intake and better academic performance than those who do not eat breakfast (Kleinman, 2002). Children who do not eat breakfast have also been found to have lower grade point averages and are absent from school more often than those who do eat breakfast (Kleinman, 2002).

Some children say they do not feel hungry at the beginning of the day, but that is usually because they have gone for months or possibly years without eating breakfast. The body adjusts the sensations of hunger and appetite based on usual eating patterns. For example, if you had a job that allowed you to eat lunch at 11 AM, you are usually hungry when 11 AM comes around. If you switch to a new job, and you are now required to take lunch at 12 PM, what happens when 11 AM comes around? More than likely you are extremely hungry. But, after a few weeks, your body adjusts and you begin to grow hungry at 12 PM. When your child does not eat breakfast, their body becomes accustomed to being deprived of energy in the morning. That does not mean that their body does not need the energy. After a week or two of eating breakfast, their body will adjust and they will have an appetite when they wake up in the morning.

Tight schedules may result in parents trying to multitask. It is convenient to stop at the corner gas station, fill up the tank, and pick up a cup of coffee for yourself and a breakfast burrito for the kids. This gets your child into the habit of eating "on-the-go" and choosing non-nutritious foods when they are in a hurry. Setting your alarm clock and waking your kids up 10 minutes earlier so that you can sit together and have breakfast will make a big difference in your child's health. Not only do they get the benefit of more nutritious foods, but they also have an opportunity to talk with other family members.

There are many options available to provide your child with a healthy breakfast, but unfortunately, there are also many unhealthy options. You should avoid breakfast foods from fast food restaurants. They are high in both fat and sodium. Some healthy breakfast options include the following:

❖ One cup of cereal (that does not have sugar listed as the first or second ingredient) with skim milk, fruit, and a glass of 100% orange juice.

❖ One or two eggs (cooked any way but fried), whole-wheat toast, fruit, and 100% orange juice.

❖ French toast, waffles, or pancakes with whole grains, fruit, and a 100% juice of any type.
❖ Oatmeal or cream of wheat with fruit, and a 100% juice of any type.
❖ English muffin or bagel made with whole grains, fruit, and a 100% juice of any type.

On the days when eating at home is completely impossible, the following can be healthy on-the-go options:

❖ A bag of dry cereal, 2 slices of whole wheat toast with a slice of low fat cheese, a hard boiled egg, a whole wheat bagel with peanut butter, or a low fat bran muffin.
❖ A 100% juice box or single serving nonfat milk.
❖ Easy to eat fruit like a banana, orange, or apple.

Bunches of Healthy Lunch

Lunchtime can be particularly challenging for parents because five days of the week your child makes choices for lunch without supervision. That is why teaching your child to make healthy choices is so important. Thankfully, many schools are beginning to recognize their responsibility for providing your child with healthy options. Vending machines that sell soft drinks are now being replaced with machines that provide water, milk, and juice. If your school still provides unhealthy meals and drinks to students, you may want to contact the school board and request that healthier choices be available to students. Some children are more likely to eat healthy if they bring their own food to school. If your child is old enough and nutritious options are available, allow them to pack their own lunch. This will allow your child to decide what foods they will be eating, and they may be more likely to eat their lunch if they choose the foods. If your child brings lunch with them to school, you can make healthy lunches by using:

❖ Whole grain breads
❖ Low sodium and low fat lunch meats, like turkey and chicken
❖ Low fat cheese
❖ Fresh fruit or a fruit cup in natural juice or light syrup
❖ Yogurt
❖ Trail mix including nuts, seeds, and dried fruit
❖ Include vegetables by placing lettuce and tomato on a sandwich or include a bag of chopped vegetables with a yogurt dip.
❖ Water, nonfat milk, or 100% juice

Winner Dinners

Whenever possible, your child should consume dinner with the family at the table. Cooking foods at home allows you to have greater control over the calories, nutrients, salt, and preparation method than eating food away from home. Many meals that you can make nutritiously at home have unnecessary additional sodium and calories when consumed in restaurants. Having meals together is beneficial for your child on many levels. You cannot be a role model for eating behaviors if your child does not see you eat. Family meals are an excellent time to discuss nutrition, such as why certain foods are good for you and why avoiding things like sodium and saturated fat are beneficial.

Getting your child involved in the process of preparing meals will help them for years to come as they learn how to prepare their own meals. Use age appropriate activities such as washing vegetables, arranging foods on a plate or platter, or stirring and mixing foods. Older children can help with cutting foods, under supervision of course.

Besides being helpful to your child's physical health, family meals are also beneficial for your child emotionally. Children have an opportunity to talk with other family members about their day, good things that happened to them, and can talk through problems they are experiencing. Due to work and other schedules, having a family meal everyday may be difficult. If that is the case, at least one meal per week should be consumed together. Family meals should take place around a table, not in front of the television. Eating meals in front of the television may lead your child to think of food every time they are watching television.

Food Prep 101

To prepare healthier meals for your family, use herbs and spices rather than salt. Removing salt all at once may be a little too dramatic of a change for your child. Decrease the amount of salt that you add to foods by one-half each week until you have eliminated salt as a seasoning. You should avoid frying as a method of cooking. Healthier options include baking, steaming, boiling, and broiling. Foods that are fried can taste just as good (if not better) when you bake them instead.

Clean the Plate No More

Do not force your child to eat everything that is on their plate at meals. Your child needs to learn to recognize the feelings of satiety and satiation. Satiety is the feeling of fullness that develops when someone is eating a meal and it stops him or her from eating more. Satiation is a feeling of fullness that a person feels between their meals. When someone overeats regularly, or allows emotions to influence food choices, they may lose the ability to recognize these signals. However, by choosing healthier foods and ending emotional eating, your child can once again learn to recognize these feelings. To avoid wasting food, place smaller portions on your child's plate. Not eating at meals becomes a problem when your child replaces meal foods with unhealthy snacks. There is no need to force a child to eat a meal if you make healthy snacks, like fruits and vegetables, available.

If you do eat out at a restaurant, the servings are typically much larger than what you or your child should consume at one sitting. This is another place where your child should not be forced to eat everything they are served. Take home leftovers and store them for another meal. Remember that these foods tend to be high in sodium, so the remainder of the intake for that day should consist of low sodium foods.

Snack Time

The snacks that children consume between meals tend to lack nutritional value. Snack foods are also usually high in calories, fat, and sodium. Children are more likely to eat fruit and vegetables as a snack if they are pre-washed and pre-cut. Place fresh fruits like bananas, apples, and oranges on the counter where your child can easily see them. Place refrigerated fruit and vegetables in clear bags. Children are more likely to eat these foods if they can see them. Place non-healthy snack foods in a location that is inconvenient such as a high cabinet. Some healthy snack ideas include:

* Make a fruit smoothie by mixing 1 cup of skim milk, ½ cup fat-free frozen yogurt, and 1 piece of fresh fruit or ½ cup of frozen fruit in a blender.
* Wash fruit as soon as you bring them home from the store so they are ready to eat when your child is looking for a snack.
* Cut up raw vegetables into small servings and provide a fat-free yogurt or dressing as dip.
* Make up small bags of unsalted nuts and dried fruit and take them with you to provide as a snack if you are away from home.

The Drink Link

Water, milk, and 100% juice are the best drinks for your child. The adequate intake for water depends on the age of your child. For children between the ages of 4 and 8, the adequate intake is 1.7 liters per day. For males between the ages of 9 and 13, 2.4 liters per day are recommended and for males between 14 and 18, 3.3 liters per day are recommended. Females between 9 and 13 need 2.1 liters per day and those between 14 and 18 need 2.3 liters per day. Males will have a higher percentage of body water than females because they have more lean tissue, or muscle.

So how much is a liter? There are about 4 and ¼ cups in a liter and one cup of fluid is equal to 8 ounces. If you are not sure how much your child is drinking, fill a glass to the level that you normally do when giving your child a drink. Then pour the fluid into a measuring cup to see how much they are consuming. The table below has the requirements in liters, cups, and ounces so you can use whichever measurement is easiest for you. These average intake requirements will change if your child is physically active because they will lose more fluid through sweat.

Liters Needed	Cups of Fluid	Ounces of fluid
1.7 liters	7.19 cups	57.52
2.1 liters	8.88	71.04
2.3 liters	9.72	77.76
2.4 liters	10.14	81.12
3.3 liters	13.95	111.6

When drinking milk, skim milk or nonfat milk is best because your child will get all of the nutrients of milk without the additional fat and calories. If your child usually consumes whole milk, slowly change from 2%, then 1%, and finally to nonfat milk. When drinking juice, 100% juice is the best option. Be careful of juices labeled as a juice "drink" or "ade." These types of juices are typically water, sugar, and very little if any actual juice. Whole fruits are better for your child than juice because your child will receive fiber when consuming the food. However, 100% juice should be limited to between 8 ounces (1 cup) and 12 ounces (1 ½ cups) per day and milk should be limited to 8 ounces (1 cup) to 16 ounces (2 cups) per day. When your child consumes more juice and milk, he or she is less likely to take in other important foods to meet their nutritional needs.

Eat Healthy, Save Money

Many people believe that it costs more money to eat healthy than to eat unhealthy, but this is not true. When the cost per serving of fruits and vegetables is considered, eating these foods can be very economical. Some fruits and vegetables are more expensive than others are, and it can depend upon whether the product is fresh, frozen, juiced, canned, or dried. Fresh fruits and vegetables may become expensive if you purchase them and they go bad before they are consumed. If this happens regularly, then purchasing frozen fruit and vegetables may be a better option for you. However, to get the most nutrients from these foods, eating fresh is best.

The following is a list of the least expensive to the most expensive fresh fruit per pound:

- ❖ Watermelon (least expensive)
- ❖ Bananas
- ❖ Grapefruit
- ❖ Cantaloupe
- ❖ Honeydew
- ❖ Oranges
- ❖ Papaya
- ❖ Mangoes
- ❖ Apples
- ❖ Pears
- ❖ Kiwi
- ❖ Tangelos
- ❖ Peaches
- ❖ Tangerines
- ❖ Nectarines
- ❖ Plums
- ❖ Grapes
- ❖ Pineapple
- ❖ Strawberries
- ❖ Apricots
- ❖ Blueberries
- ❖ Cherries
- ❖ Raspberries
- ❖ Blackberries (most expensive)

The following is a list of the least expensive to the most expensive fresh vegetables per pound:

- ❖ Potatoes (least expensive)

❖ Cabbage
❖ Whole carrots
❖ Onions
❖ Sweet potatoes
❖ Cucumbers
❖ Iceberg lettuce
❖ Celery
❖ Radishes
❖ Sweet corn
❖ Broccoli
❖ Eggplant
❖ Broccoli fleurets
❖ Plum tomatoes
❖ Leaf lettuce
❖ Green beans
❖ Cauliflower
❖ Bell peppers
❖ Romaine lettuce
❖ Regular tomatoes
❖ Brussels sprouts
❖ Baby carrots
❖ Spinach
❖ Zucchini squash
❖ Cauliflower fleurets
❖ Kale
❖ Mustard Greens
❖ Asparagus
❖ Turnip greens
❖ Okra
❖ Green peas
❖ Cherry tomatoes
❖ Whole mushrooms
❖ Collard greens
❖ Sliced mushrooms (most expensive)

*Source: United States Department of Agriculture. How much do Americans pay for fruits and vegetables/AIB-790. Economic Research Service. www.ers.usda.gov/publications/aib790/aib790f.pdf

The most and least expensive ways to buy and eat fruit depends upon the type of fruit. When you consider the cost per pound or pint, blackberries, raspberries, pineapple, and apples are the most expensive when purchased fresh. Blackberries and raspberries are the cheapest when purchased canned. Pineapples and apples are the least expensive when purchased as unsweetened juice. Fresh is the cheapest way to purchase papaya, mango, pears, blueberries, and cherries. Peaches or apricots packed in juice and strawberries are the least expensive when purchased canned. (USDA, 2007)

Vegetables also differ in their cost depending upon whether they are fresh, frozen, or canned. Per pound, fresh is the most expensive and canned is the least expensive way to purchase collard greens, green peas, okra, turnip greens, mustard greens, kale, and spinach. Fresh is the cheapest way to purchase potatoes, green cabbage, sweet potatoes, broccoli, cauliflower, and Brussels sprouts. (USDA, 2007)

Many people believe that eating from a fast food restaurant is cheaper than purchasing foods in a grocery store and cooking foods at home. If a family of four went to a fast food restaurant and ate three items that cost one dollar each (an egg/chicken/fish sandwich or hamburger, drink, and one side) for all three meals a day for one week it would cost $252.00. On the other hand, a family of four with two children between the ages of 6 and 11 who eat their meals and snacks at home would spend considerably less. The United States Department of Agriculture has determined how much families spend when following a thrifty, low-cost, moderate-cost, and liberal shopping plan. Following the thrifty plan, a family of four would spend $123.10. For the low-cost plan, the cost is $157.30, for the moderate-cost $195.80, and for the liberal plan $237.70 (USDA, 2007). Eating at a fast food restaurant is more expensive than the most liberal shopping plan. Consider that not everything that most people consume from a fast food restaurant comes from the dollar menu and the cost increases even more.

Stay Safe in the Kitchen

Healthy foods provide great nutrition to your child, but you also need to keep foods safe to eat. You should wash fruits and vegetables thoroughly before you and your children consume them. A great way to ensure that fruits and vegetables are clean is to wash them as soon as you bring them home. You should scrub these foods with a fruit and vegetable brush to remove any left-over chemicals that might be on the surface of the food.

Make sure counter tops and cutting surfaces are clean when cutting up fresh fruits and vegetables. Clean surfaces with a disinfectant after cutting up meat products. Avoid using wooden cutting boards because cuts that are left in the wood may fill with bacteria that are difficult to remove and can contaminate other foods placed on the same surface.

You need to cook meat, poultry, and fish to certain temperatures to ensure these foods are safe to eat. The temperature required depends upon the type of food you are cooking. You should cook whole turkey, chicken, duck, goose, and poultry thighs to a temperature of 180°F (USDA). Poultry breasts and well-done beef, veal, lamb, or pork need to reach a temperature of 170°F (USDA). Turkey or chicken ground meat and stuffing require a temperature of 165°F (USDA).Veal, beef, lamb, or pork ground meat and medium-done fresh beef, veal, lamb of pork should be cooked to 160°F (USDA). You should cook fish until it is white and flakes with a fork (USDA).

Summary Points

* ❖ *The principles of variety and moderation should be used when choosing foods.*
* ❖ *It is necessary for your child to eat at least 3 healthy meals per day, preferably 4-5 small meals.*
* ❖ *Breakfast affects academic performance and nutrient intake.*
* ❖ *Children who do not typically eat upon awakening can learn to enjoy breakfast.*
* ❖ *Lunches supplied by schools should be healthy.*
* ❖ *Healthy options are available when making lunch for your child to eat at school.*
* ❖ *Family meals allow your child to observe role models, discuss nutrition, and talk about their day.*
* ❖ *Prepare foods with herbs and spices rather than salt.*
* ❖ *Bake, steam, boil, and broil rather than fry.*
* ❖ *Do not force your child to eat everything that is on their plate.*
* ❖ *Snacks should be low in calories, fat, and sodium.*
* ❖ *Water, milk, and 100% juice are the best drinks for your child.*
* ❖ *Too much milk and juice may prevent your child from taking in other nutritious foods.*
* ❖ *Eating healthy does not cost more than eating unhealthy.*
* ❖ *Eating at fast food restaurants is more expensive than buying foods from a grocery store.*
* ❖ *Foods can be kept safe to eat by washing, cutting, and cooking properly.*

CHAPTER 5

WHEN GOOD FOODS GO BAD

There are certain foods that should be limited in your child's diet. Foods that are high in saturated fat, trans fat, and high in sodium, foods that provide empty calories, and fast foods should be limited, and will be referred to as "limiting foods". These foods will have negative effects on your child's health when consumed excessively. When your child consumes "limiting foods" on a regular basis, your child is less likely to take in other more nutritious foods. A great overall rule when deciding what foods to limit in your child's diet is to increase their intake of foods made outside (fruits, vegetables, seeds, nuts, etc.) and decrease their intake of foods made inside (processed foods, fast foods, junk foods, etc.)

You should not eliminate these foods from your child's diet because children should be allowed to have cake or ice cream at a celebration or have chips and soda at a family picnic. Not allowing these types of foods during special occasions may lead your child to feel deprived and they may try to sneak these foods. This can contribute to an unhealthy emotional relationship with food (See Chapter 8).

Bad Fats

There are several types of fats including polyunsaturated, monounsaturated, saturated, and trans fats. Polyunsaturated and monounsaturated fats are an important part of your child's diet. They provide Omega-3 and Omega-6 fatty acids that are essential for the proper growth and development of your child. On the other hand, foods that are high in saturated fat and trans fat can contribute to the development of high cholesterol levels and increase the risk for heart disease. Saturated and trans fats should be limited in your child's diet.

You should also read the ingredient list of a food and avoid those that contain hydrogenated oils. When oils and other fats are hydrogenated, they have been converted from polyunsaturated or monounsaturated fats to saturated fats. In other words, they are changed from the fats that are good for you to the fats that are bad for you. Why would a manufacturer do that? Because saturated fats, such as hydrogenated oils, do not go bad as quickly, so the food stays stable for a longer time. This process also changes a fat from a liquid to a solid, which is used to make some types of margarine. Just like saturated fats, hydrogenated fats are bad for the health of the heart. Foods that have been hydrogenated are typically high in trans fats. Some ways to decrease your child's intake of these fats include the following:

❖ Decrease the use of red meat and increase the use of skinless poultry and fish.
❖ If red meat is consumed, choose lean meats and cutoff visible fat before cooking.
❖ Limit the intake of fried foods. Bake, steam, boil, or broil foods instead.
❖ When purchasing processed foods, read the food label and avoid purchasing those that contain more than 0.5 grams of saturated fat or those that contain any trans fats.
❖ Use nonfat or low fat milk rather than whole milk (1% milk has 1.5 grams of saturated fat for 1 cup as opposed to 4.6 grams of saturated fat for whole milk).
❖ Substitute low fat cheese for those made with whole milk.
❖ Use sherbet as a treat rather than ice cream.
❖ Limit cookies, cakes, and pastries.
❖ Avoid coconut oil, palm oil, palm kernel oil, and cocoa butter. Use safflower, sesame, canola, and olive oils instead.

Bad Calories

Foods and drinks that provide empty calories in your child's diet should be limited. Empty calorie foods and drinks are those that provide the body with calories but do not provide other beneficial nutrients. Examples include candy, cookies, junk foods, and soft drinks. Because these products provide energy, your child will be less likely to take in fruits, vegetables, and other nutritious foods.

Candy, cookies, and other cake products provide a large amount of simple sugars and tend to be high in saturated fat. Because these products contain many simple sugars, they cause the blood sugar to increase quickly. This usually provides the person who consumes these products with a burst of energy. However, after this initial burst of energy comes the "crash". The energy "crash" occurs when your child becomes tired and sleepy and your child may turn to another empty calorie source to provide an additional surge of energy. Sugars that come from fruit are released more slowly into the blood stream. Because of this, they provide a steady release of energy rather than a surge and crash. Some ways to decrease your child's intake of foods that can cause an energy crash include:

❖ Offer a piece of fruit or a fruit smoothie when your child is craving something sweet.
❖ If your child consumes a large number of cookies, candy, or cake, decrease the number they take in by one piece or slice every four days.
❖ Introduce fruit as an alternate to other sweets by substituting a piece of candy, a cookie, or slice of cake with a piece of fruit.

Other "junk foods" like chips should also be limited. These foods can be high in saturated fat, trans fat, and sodium. Slowly decreasing your child's intake of these foods will benefit their health. You can start by making healthier substitutions for the junk foods that your child consumes. For example:

❖ Substitute potato chips with baked chips.
❖ Substitute pretzels for chips.
❖ Purchase those that come in single serving packages to prevent excessive consumption.

However, it is best that your child does not consume junk foods on a daily basis. After switching to the healthier options, start to decrease the number of these foods by ½ per week. For example, if your child usually has potato chips 2 times a day, cut it down to 1 or decrease the amount they consume at those two sittings by one half. Keep reducing the amount by ½ until your child in not eating junk foods on a daily basis.

What ever you call them, soft drinks, soda, or pop, these drinks add unnecessary additional calories, sugar, caffeine, and sodium to your child's intake. If your child drinks a lot of soft drinks, decrease the number they drink by one soda per week. Your child should consume soft drinks only on occasion (if at all). Substitute soda with water, milk, or 100% juice.

Bad Salt

Sodium is a very important mineral in the body. As you will learn in the vitamin and mineral chapter, sodium is necessary for maintaining a balance of fluid in the body and for muscle contraction. However, when sodium is consumed in amounts greater than what the body requires, it can cause the blood pressure to increase and the heart must work harder to do its job. This can increase your child's risk for heart disease as they age. A high sodium intake can increase your child's risk of developing osteoporosis as they age because with an increase in sodium intake there is also an increase in the loss of calcium from the body.

Sodium is found in the highest amounts in processed foods because it is added as a preservative by those who manufacture the food. Sodium is also found naturally in foods such as meat, poultry, and milk. Naturally occurring sodium is usually present in much smaller amounts than sodium found in processed foods. To limit the amount of sodium in your child's diet, try the following:

- ❖ Limit your child's intake of fast food.
- ❖ Limit your child's intake of processed foods, including bacon, sausage, and ham.
- ❖ Limit your child's intake of canned soup and canned meat or fish. If canned tuna is purchased, those packed in water are the best option to decrease sodium.
- ❖ Limit and eventually eliminate the use of table salt.
- ❖ Increase your child's intake of fresh fruits and vegetables.

Fresh fruits and vegetables are best, but you can also purchase frozen vegetables. Vegetables that are canned are often high in sodium, so make sure you check the food label. Rinsing canned vegetables will remove some sodium, but other nutrients will also be lost. Processed meats are also often very high in sodium. If you purchase meat from a deli counter, ask them how much sodium is in a serving of the meat before you purchase the product. If you purchase pre-cut meat in a package, read the food label. If your child is used to adding extra salt to their foods from the saltshaker, slowly start to decrease the amount of salt your child adds by ¼ of a teaspoon per week until table salt is no longer used. It will take some time, but eventually your child will become accustomed to eating foods without adding salt and they will become sensitive to foods with a high salt intake.

For children that are between the ages of 6 and 8, no more than 1,900 mg of sodium should be consumed daily. For those older than 9, no more than 2,300 mg should be consumed daily. It is important to pay attention to food labels to see how much sodium is in a serving of a food. Limit your child's intake of foods that have more than 140 mg of sodium per serving.

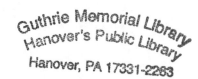

Bad Fast Foods

Fast foods should be limited as much as possible in your child's diet. Your child should eat foods from a fast food restaurant no more than once a week, preferably no more than once a month. These foods tend to be high in saturated and trans fats and have little nutrients. Fast foods are also high in sodium, so they can contribute to high blood pressure as well as heart disease.

Fast food establishments are like any other business, their goal is to draw you in and keep you coming back as often as possible. They target your child by offering toys related to the most popular cartoon character or movie at that time. Unfortunately, along with the toy, most fast food restaurants also offer up foods that lead to poor health. Thankfully, fast food restaurants are now offering healthier choices, especially for kids.

At some of the most popular fast food restaurants, one meal can provide your child with more calories than they should consume in an entire day. Let's say, for example, you take your child to Burger King® and your child orders a Whopper with cheese (760 calories), large French fries (500 calories), an apple pie (300 calories), and a medium 22 ounce Coke (200 calories). That would be **1,760** calories-for one meal! By the way, that meal would also provide your child with 2,410 mg of sodium. That is more than the recommended maximum sodium intake for an entire day for those 9 and older. Do you think a fish filet sandwich or a chicken sandwich would be better? Not by much! The fish filet sandwich is 660 calories and the chicken sandwich is 583 calories. Your child has consumed all those calories and received very little nutrients. (Burger King® Nutrition)

How about McDonald's® for breakfast? McDonald's® hotcakes and sausage provide 780 calories, 33 grams of fat, and 1,020 mg of sodium (McDonald's USA Nutritional Information). A great learning opportunity for you and your child is to get on the computer before you go to a fast food restaurant. All fast food restaurants have the nutritional information for their foods online. Go to the website with your child before you leave the house. Look up the calorie, fat, and sodium content of the different foods and make a decision of what to eat before you go to the fast food establishment. The following is a list of website address for several fast food places so that you can look up nutritional content:

Arby's™: http://www.arbys.com
Burger King®: http://www.bk.com
Domino's®: http://www.dominos.com/home/index.jsp
Kentucky Fried Chicken®: http://www.kfc.com/
Long John Silver's™: http://www.ljsilvers.com

McDonald's®: http://www.mcdonalds.com/usa.html
Papa John's™: http://www.papajohns.com/
Pizza Hut®: http://www.pizzahut.com/
Subway®: http://www.subway.com/subwayroot/index.aspx
Taco Bell®: http://www.tacobell.com/
Wendy's®: http://www.wendys.com

The "healthy" choices at fast food restaurants can often be unexpectedly high in fat and calories. Salads can actually be higher in calories than hamburgers if there is fried chicken, bacon, or high fat dressing added. The following are some ways to make eating at a fast food restaurant healthier:

❖ Look up nutritional information before going to a fast food restaurant.

❖ When you take your child to a fast food restaurant, resist the temptation to get the most for your money. It is often hard to pass up on increasing a portion size for a few extra cents. Buying the smaller serving will make a big difference in the amount of calories your child consumes.

Rewards

The rewards system can be used when your child chooses healthy foods as well as when your child chooses not to consume the "limiting foods". For example, they may choose to drink one less soda, choose a fruit or vegetable as a snack over cookies, or choose a healthy option at a fast food restaurant for an additional star on the rewards chart. They can also receive a star when they decide not to add extra salt to their food.

Real Life Lesson

I always enjoy seeing how on the first night of my college nutrition class, students arrive with their soda bottles and coffee cups; but a few weeks into the semester they begin arriving with water and juice instead. One of my students, I will call her Mary, approached me several weeks into the class. Mary told me that she, her husband, and her 8 and 10-year-old daughters ate fast food at least 4 times a week and drank soda all day long, even at breakfast. She said that at her husband's last doctor visit, his cholesterol was over 280 and he was placed on cholesterol lowering medication. Everyone in the family was overweight and Mary was concerned about her family's health. She told me that her family was going to cut back on their soda and fast food intake.

The end of the semester came and after the final exam, Mary told me that her family was resistant at first, but that they only had fast food once in the last month and that she eliminated all soda from her house. To be honest, after several semesters I had forgotten about Mary's story. One year later, I received an e-mail from Mary. She told me that everyone in the family had lost weight and that her husband and 8-year-old daughter were now a healthy weight.

She said she couldn't believe how much more energy she had and that she could think more clearly when studying. Her husband's cholesterol level came down 60 points thanks to the dietary changes and medication. Her daughters were not tired all the time and the whole family started being more active. She said her kids looked healthier and happy and started performing better in school. She repeatedly thanked me, but I pointed out to her that I only provided her with the information; she was the one who took the information and created a better life for her family. That is what I am doing with this book, giving you the information so that you can make the difference in your child's life.

Summary Points

- ❖ *Increase your child's intake of foods made outside and decrease your child's intake of foods made outside.*
- ❖ *Polyunsaturated and monounsaturated fats are important to good health.*
- ❖ *Saturated and trans fats should be limited because they increase the risk of heart disease.*
- ❖ *Foods that contain hydrogenated oils should be limited in your child's diet.*
- ❖ *Foods that provide empty calories including cookies, cake products, junk foods, and soda should be limited.*
- ❖ *Sodium should be limited because excessive intake increases the blood pressure and increases the risk for heart disease as well as osteoporosis.*
- ❖ *Fast foods should be limited because they are high in saturated and trans fats and provide little nutrients.*
- ❖ *The rewards system can be used to encourage your child to decrease their intake of the limiting foods.*

CHAPTER 6

VITAMINS AND MINERALS

Vitamins and minerals are very important to your child's good health. Following the plan outlined in this book will help your child receive vitamins and minerals from the foods your child consumes. In particular, eating fruits and vegetables will aid in meeting these needs. It is important for your child to receive nutrients from fruits and vegetables and not to rely on supplements to meet their needs. There are other materials contained in these food products that are beneficial to your child's health. However, a multivitamin and multimineral supplement will also be beneficial. Most people refer to multivitamins and multiminerals by as "vitamin supplements", so this term will be used from now on in this book.

Vitamins do not provide the body with energy, but they help the body use energy from carbohydrates, fats, and proteins. Without vitamins, your body cannot effectively receive energy from these other foods. When some adults take vitamin supplements, they choose to take each one separately rather then in a multivitamin or multimineral supplement. This is dangerous for adults to do, but presents an even greater danger for children. It is possible that you will supplement too much of a vitamin leading to toxic amounts in the body. With vitamins and minerals, some people think if a little is good, a lot must be better. This is *not* true. Toxic levels of vitamins can cause health problems, just as deficiencies can. So, using a vitamin supplement that is created for children is the best option.

For younger children, there are commercially available chewable vitamin supplements that have a taste that children like, and most parents are met with little resistance when asking children to take them. As your child gets older, you can switch to vitamin supplements that your child can swallow. These vitamin supplements typically have higher amounts of vitamins and minerals to meet an older child's needs. However, a chewable vitamin is better than none at all if your child will not swallow pill forms.

CAUTION: Please do not refer to vitamin supplements as candy or use products that look very similar to candy. There are now vitamins that look like gum balls or gummy bears. When you are not around, your child may get a hold of the vitamins and eat several because they look, and taste, just like candy. This can lead to toxic levels of vitamins and minerals in your child. If this does happen, immediately contact the poison control center in your state for further instructions and information.

In the tables that I will provide you, which list the amount of vitamins and minerals that are recommended based on the age of your child, some have a star and say "Adequate Intake." Adequate Intake is something that is set for a nutrient when there is no recommended daily allowance (RDA). The RDA is determined after tests have been performed to figure out how much of the vitamins and minerals children and adults need. When those tests have not been performed, an Adequate Intake level is set instead. The tables of vitamins and minerals also have "upper intake levels" listed. When I list symptoms of excessive intake, these symptoms may begin to develop if intake of the vitamin or mineral is above the upper intake level. If the upper intake level is blank on the table, it means that upper intake levels have not been determined for that vitamin or mineral.

Types of Vitamins

There are two types of vitamins, water-soluble and fat-soluble. The body filters out the water-soluble vitamins on a regular basis and they need to be replenished nearly every day. Water-soluble vitamins include the B vitamins and vitamin C. The fat-soluble vitamins are stored in the body's fat, and do not need to be replenished as often. The fat-soluble vitamins include vitamins A, D, E, and K. Two of the fat-soluble vitamins can also be made by the body. Vitamin D is created when the skin is exposed to sun light and natural bacteria that are present in the intestines create vitamin K. Excessive intakes of the fat-soluble vitamins are more likely to cause toxicity than the water-soluble vitamins. If your child's kidneys are healthy, the water-soluble vitamins are filtered out of the blood. Because the fat-soluble vitamins are stored in the body's fat, the risk of being deficient decreases and the risk of having excessive amounts through supplements increases.

Water-Soluble Vitamins

The B vitamins include vitamins B_1, B_2, B_3, B_5, B_6, B_7, B_9, and B_{12}. Vitamin B_1 is also known as thiamin and is needed in the body to break down carbohydrates and proteins. It is required to allow the nerve and muscle cells to function correctly. You can find thiamin in enriched grain, bread, and cereal products, organ meats, and legumes. If the body becomes deficient of thiamin, loss of appetite, tiredness, irritability, and constipation may be experienced. Severe deficiency can cause a disease called beriberi where the muscles begin to weaken and waste away. Consuming too much thiamin has not been shown to cause problems.

Riboflavin (B_2) aids enzymes found in the body and allows them to work properly to break down carbohydrates, fats, and proteins. You can find riboflavin in enriched grain products as well as milk, organ meats, meat, poultry, and fish. Too little riboflavin can cause itching and burning of the eyes and cracks around the mouth. Just like thiamin, consuming too much riboflavin has not been shown to cause toxic reactions.

Vitamin B_3 is niacin, and is needed in order to obtain energy from carbohydrates, fats, and proteins. It can be found in protein sources (meat, poultry, and fish) and enriched bread products. If the body does not have enough niacin, it can cause weakness, irritability, and anxiety. A severe deficiency can cause the disease pellagra with confusion, skin sores, and poor memory. A deficiency is usually not a problem because most people consume more meat products than they really need. If too much niacin is consumed, it can cause a niacin flush. The skin becomes red, tingly, painful, and itchy. When high levels of niacin are consumed regularly, it can affect the functioning of the liver.

Pantothenic acid, also known as vitamin B_5, is used to break down carbohydrates, fats, and proteins. You can find pantothenic acid in grains, animal products including chicken and fish, and some vegetables such as broccoli and tomatoes. It is rare for someone to have too little B_5, but if it were to occur it could cause weakness and tiredness. There are no known side effects of consuming too much pantothenic acid.

Vitamin B_6 is needed to break down proteins that are consumed and can be found in fortified products, organ meats, poultry, fish, and some fruits and vegetables. A deficiency is rare, but can cause weakness, dizziness, and depression. Consuming too much B_6 is not known to cause any problems.

Biotin is needed in the body to make body proteins and to store blood sugar. Small amounts of biotin are found in meats, eggs, and fruits. The natural bacteria that are located in the intestines can also create biotin. Since the body's bacteria create it, if someone is on antibiotics for a long period of time a deficiency can develop. The usual length of antibiotic therapy, from 5 to 14 days, is typically not enough to cause a deficiency. There are no known side effects from consuming too much biotin.

Folic Acid, or Folate, is particularly important for growing children because it is needed for cells that are rapidly dividing. Most bread and cereal products have been enriched with folic acid to prevent deficiencies in pregnant women. Just as a growing baby needs this vitamin to develop correctly, children need the vitamin as they continue to grow and develop. You can also find this vitamin in dark green leafy vegetables. Folic acid and vitamin B_{12} work together to help prevent a certain type of anemia. Vitamin B_{12} helps to protect nerve cells and red blood cells. You can find B_{12} in meat, poultry, and fish, as well as products that are fortified with the vitamin. A deficiency of folic acid and B_{12} can cause anemia.

Vitamin B_{12} and folic acid are one example of why it is better to use a multivitamin supplement rather than supplementing each vitamin individually. For example, let's say you choose to supplement each vitamin individually and you gave your child a folic acid supplement and not a B_{12} supplement. The folic acid would mask all the symptoms of a B_{12} deficiency until the late stages. Why is that dangerous? If there is too little B_{12} and it is not caught until the late stages, it can cause damage to the body's nervous system.

The last water-soluble vitamin is vitamin C, which is an antioxidant in the body and helps the body heal when there is an injury. Antioxidants protect the body from damage. When most people think of vitamin C, they think of citrus fruits. Citrus fruits are a good source of the vitamin, but other great sources include strawberries, bell peppers, and broccoli. Vitamin C is destroyed when it is exposed to high temperatures and cooking, so only raw fruits and vegetables would be a good source. Too little vitamin C can interfere with healing from an injury, and can cause bruising and bleeding to occur more easily. If the body is deficient for a long time, the disease scurvy can develop, which affects the muscles and the nervous system. You only need small amounts of vitamin C to prevent this disease. Too much vitamin C can cause diarrhea and nausea.

If your child has anemia and needs to increase their iron intake, it is helpful to include a food that is high in vitamin C with one that is high in iron. The acid in vitamin C helps the body absorb iron. So, at dinner if you feed your child a meat product (high in iron) with broccoli (high in vitamin C) it would help your child absorb the iron.

Water Soluble Vitamins	Recommended Daily Allowance (RDA) or Adequate Intake		Upper Intake Level
Thiamin (B$_1$)	Children 4-8 years:	0.6 mg	
	Children 9-13 years:	0.9 mg	
	Males 14-18 years:	1.2 mg	
	Females 14-18 years:	1.0 mg	
Riboflavin (B$_2$)	Children 4-8 years:	0.6 mg	
	Children 9-13 years:	0.9 mg	
	Males 14-18 years:	1.3 mg	
	Females 14-18 years:	1.0 mg	
Niacin (B$_3$)	Children 4-8 years:	8 mg	15 mg
	Children 9-13 years:	12 mg	20 mg
	Males 14-18 years:	16 mg	30 mg
	Females 14-18 years:	14 mg	30 mg
Pantothenic Acid (B$_5$) * Adequate Intake not RDA	Children 4-8 years:	3 mg	
	Children 9-13 years:	4 mg	
	Males 14-18 years:	5 mg	
	Females 14-18 years:	5 mg	
Vitamin B$_6$	Children 4-8 years:	0.6 mg	40 mg
	Children 9-13 years:	1.0 mg	60 mg
	Males 14-18 years:	1.3 mg	80 mg
	Females 14-18 years:	1.2 mg	80 mg
Biotin (B$_7$) * Adequate Intake not RDA	Children 4-8 years:	12 mg	
	Children 9-13 years:	20 mg	
	Males 14-18 years:	25 mg	
	Females 14-18 years:	25 mg	
Folate, Folic Acid (B$_9$)	Children 4-8 years:	200 mcg	400 mcg
	Children 9-13 years:	300 mcg	600 mcg
	Males 14-18 years:	400 mcg	800 mcg
	Females 14-18 years:	400 mcg	800 mcg

Water Soluble Vitamins	Recommended Daily Allowance (RDA) or Adequate Intake		Upper Intake Level
Vitamin B$_{12}$ (Cobalamin)	Children 4-8 years:	1.2 mcg	
	Children 9-13 years:	1.8 mcg	
	Males 14-18 years:	2.4 mcg	
	Females 14-18 years:	2.4 mcg	
Vitamin C	Children 4-8 years:	25 mg	650 mg
	Children 9-13 years:	45 mg	1,200 mg
	Males 14-18 years:	75 mg	1,800 mg
	Females 14-18 years:	65 mg	1,800 mg

* Source: Dietary Reference Intakes (DRIs): Recommended Intakes for Individuals, Vitamins. *Food and Nutrition Board, Institute of Medicine, National Academies.* www.iom.edu

Fat-Soluble Vitamins

As mentioned earlier, the fat-soluble vitamins include A, D, E, and K. Vitamin A has many roles in the body including maintaining vision and growth, and it acts like a hormone in the body. Sources include animal products like fish, dairy products like milk and butter, and dark fruits and vegetables. Too little vitamin A can cause night blindness, rough skin, damage to the eyes, and decreases the body's ability to fight infection. If too much vitamin A is consumed from supplements, it can result in hair loss, headaches, nausea, bone pain, and liver problems.

Plants have a form of vitamin A called beta-carotene. Because this is a fat-soluble vitamin, it is stored in the fat underneath the skin. When your child eats many vegetables that are high in beta-carotene, like carrots or spinach, their skin can become orange or yellow in color. Cutting back on the amount of foods they are eating that are high in beta-carotene for a few days will cause this discoloration to disappear.

Vitamin D is very important to the development of the bones and can be made by the skin from exposure to sun light. It is not possible to overdose on vitamin D through sun exposure. When your body reaches the necessary amount of the vitamin, further production stops. The use of sunscreen of SPF 8 or above prevents the skin from creating vitamin D. Only 10-15 minutes of sun exposure are needed 2-3 days per week. Of course, most parents are also concerned about skin cancer. Depending on where you live, taking your child out during the peak heat of the sun can cause sunburn in only 10-15 minutes. So, it is better to choose times when the unprotected exposure will not cause burns, after the 10-15 minutes, sunscreen can be applied.

People who live in Northern states with long cloudy winters or cities with smog or air pollution issues may develop a deficiency due to decreased sun exposure. Milk that is fortified with vitamin D is an excellent dietary source of the vitamin. Other dietary sources include fish, liver, and eggs. If your child does not drink milk or get adequate sun exposure, then supplements may be necessary, but check with your child's health care provider first. If the body has too little vitamin D, a disease called rickets can develop, which results in bowing of the arms and legs. If someone consumes excessive amounts of vitamin D by taking supplements (more than 50 micrograms per day), it can cause nausea, vomiting, kidney and heart problems, and weakness.

Like vitamin C, vitamin E is an antioxidant in the body and helps to protect against cell damage. You can find vitamin E in many foods including leafy green vegetables, nuts, whole grains, eggs, fruit, and meats. A deficiency of vitamin E usually occurs only if someone has a problem absorbing the vitamin. If a deficiency were to develop, it could cause problems with the neurological system in children. Side effects from consuming too much vitamin E are rare, but it can interfere with the body's ability to clot the blood.

The last of the fat-soluble vitamins is vitamin K, which the body needs to clot the blood and is involved in creating proteins. The natural bacteria that are present in the intestines make this vitamin. As was mentioned under the water-soluble vitamin biotin, if your child is on antibiotics, in addition to killing the bad bacteria, antibiotics may also kill the good bacteria that are present in the intestines. There are now supplements of what are called "probiotics" that can be used to replace these natural bacteria. The bacteria that are present in yogurt can also be a way to replace these bacteria while on antibiotics. You can also find vitamin K in leafy green vegetables. A deficiency of vitamin K can interfere with blood clotting, and if too much vitamin K is consumed from supplements, it can cause anemia.

Fat Soluble Vitamins	Recommended Daily Allowance (RDA) or Adequate Intake		Upper Intake Level
Vitamin A	Children 4-8 years:	400 mcg	900 mcg
	Children 9-13 years:	600 mcg	1,700 mcg
	Males 14-18 years:	900 mcg	2,800 mcg
	Females 14-18 years:	700 mcg	2,800 mcg
Vitamin D *Adequate Intake not RDA	Children 4-8 years:	5 mcg	50 mcg
	Children 9-13 years:	5 mcg	50 mcg
	Males 14-18 years:	5 mcg	50 mcg
	Females 14-18 years:	5 mcg	50 mcg
Vitamin E	Children 4-8 years:	7 mg	300 mg
	Children 9-13 years:	11 mg	600 mg
	Males 14-18 years:	15 mg	800 mg
	Females 14-18 years:	15 mg	800 mg
Vitamin K *Adequate Intake not RDA	Children 4-8 years:	55 mcg	
	Children 9-13 years:	60 mcg	
	Males 14-18 years:	75 mcg	
	Females 14-18 years:	75 mcg	

* Source: Dietary Reference Intakes (DRIs): Recommended Intakes for Individuals, Vitamins. *Food and Nutrition Board, Institute of Medicine, National Academies.* www.iom.edu

Minerals

There are two types of minerals, the major minerals and the trace minerals. The only difference between the two types is the amount that is present in the body. The major minerals are found in large quantities and the trace minerals are found in smaller quantities. However, both types of minerals are extremely important to the growth and development of your child. The major minerals include calcium, magnesium, phosphorus, potassium, and sodium. The trace minerals include chromium, copper, fluoride, iodine, iron, manganese, molybdenum, selenium, and zinc.

Major Minerals

It is very important that your child receive enough calcium during their growing years. Most people know how important calcium is for the bones, but did you know that if your blood does not have enough calcium it will actually take it from the bones? The calcium that is in the blood is responsible for muscle contractions, including the beating of the heart, and for the functioning of the nervous system. Although a very small percent of the body's calcium is in the blood, it plays such an important role that the body will take more from the bones if the blood levels become low. That is why eating foods high in calcium is so important; it prevents your body from turning to the bones as a source of the mineral. If the body continuously draws calcium from the bones, it increases the risk of osteoporosis and bone fractures later in life. The best source of calcium is dairy products, including milk, cheese, and yogurt. Other sources include tofu products, nuts, fortified breads, and leafy green vegetables. Too much calcium can cause nausea, vomiting, muscle weakness, and can lead to kidney stones.

Chloride is found in processed foods, usually along with sodium. It can also be found in table salt, milk, meat, eggs, and cheese. Chloride is a part of the acid in the stomach that helps the body digest foods. It also maintains a balance of body fluids. Low levels of chloride can cause tiredness and nausea. High levels of chloride can cause the blood pressure to increase.

Magnesium is needed for the development of the bones, allows the heart to beat normally, allows the immune system to function properly, and helps to maintain blood sugar levels. This mineral can be found in leafy green vegetables, nuts, meats, legumes, bananas, and whole grains. If a deficiency of magnesium develops, it can result in heart, and muscular problems and disorientation. Too much magnesium can cause nausea, vomiting, and muscle weakness.

Phosphorus is needed for proper bone and teeth development, to break down carbohydrates, fats, and proteins, and is required to use vitamins that are consumed. It can be found in milk, cheese, yogurt, meat, eggs, cereals, nuts, legumes, and breads. If the body does not have enough phosphorus, it can result in malformed bones and teeth, weakened muscles, tiredness, and can interfere with growth. Too much phosphorus can cause anemia, diarrhea, arthritis, and can interfere with the absorption of calcium and magnesium.

Potassium is found in fresh fruits and vegetables, legumes, meats, and dairy products. It is needed for contraction of the muscles, maintaining a balance of fluids in the body, and for the functioning of the nervous system. Too little potassium can affect mental functioning, the muscles, and the heart. High levels of potassium are only a concern from supplements, not from food sources.

If too much potassium is taken in through supplements, it can cause irregular heartbeats.

Sodium allows the cells to function normally and helps to maintain a balance of fluids in the body. Sodium is found in the highest quantities in processed foods. Because there is so much sodium in our diets, it is typically not added to vitamin supplements. If the body does not have enough sodium, it can result in nausea, tiredness, and muscle cramps. High levels of sodium can cause the blood pressure to increase and if consumed on a regular basis, increases the risk of cardiovascular disease.

Major Minerals	Recommended Daily Allowance (RDA) or Adequate Intake		Upper Intake Level
Calcium *Adequate Intake not RDA	Children 4-8 years:	800 mg	2,500 mg
	Children 9-13 years:	1,300 mg	2,500 mg
	Males 14-18 years:	1,300 mg	2,500 mg
	Females 14-18 years:	1,300 mg	2,500 mg
Chloride *Adequate Intake not RDA	Children 4-8 years:	1,900 mg	2,900 mg
	Children 9-13 years:	2,300 mg	3,400 mg
	Males 14-18 years:	2,300 mg	3,600 mg
	Females 14-18 years:	2,300 mg	3,600 mg
Magnesium	Children 4-8 years:	130 mg	
	Children 9-13 years:	240 mg	350 mg
	Males 14-18 years:	410 mg	350 mg
	Females 14-18 years:	360 mg	350 mg
Phosphorus	Children 4-8 years:	500 mg	3,000 mg
	Children 9-13 years:	1,250 mg	4,000 mg
	Males 14-18 years:	1,250 mg	4,000 mg
	Females 14-18 years:	1,250 mg	4,000 mg
Potassium *Adequate Intake not RDA	Children 4-8 years:	3,800 mg	
	Children 9-13 years:	4,500 mg	
	Males 14-18 years:	4,700 mg	
	Females 14-18 years:	4,700 mg	

Sodium	Children 4-8 years:	1,200 mg	1,900 mg
*Adequate Intake not RDA	Children 9-13 years:	1,500 mg	2,200 mg
	Males 14-18 years:	1,500 mg	2,300 mg
	Females 14-18 years:	1,500 mg	2,300 mg

* Source: Dietary Reference Intakes (DRIs): Recommended Intakes for Individuals, Elements. *Food and Nutrition Board, Institute of Medicine, National Academies.* www.iom.edu

Trace Minerals

Chromium is found in vegetable oils, meat, poultry, and fish and helps to control blood sugar levels. Too little chromium can result in problems with the breakdown of blood sugar and too much can result in kidney problems. Copper is required by the body to form red blood cells and is needed to heal wounds. This mineral can be found in organ meats, seafood, nuts, seeds, and grains. Low levels of copper can interfere with growth and may cause anemia. Too much copper can cause vomiting, diarrhea, and liver problems.

Fluoride is needed to help form the bones and the teeth, and it helps protect the teeth from cavities. Fluoride can be found in fluorinated drinking water, fish, and fluorinated dental products. Before supplementing fluoride, it is important to find out if you have fluorinated drinking water or if your child's school has a fluoride program. If your child is receiving the mineral from school or through drinking water, do *not* use additional supplements unless directed by your child's health care provider. Too much fluoride is actually bad for the teeth and can cause pitting and staining of the enamel. For children between the ages of 4 and 8, they should not consume more than 2.2 milligrams per day and for children between 9 and 18 they should not consume more than 10 milligrams per day.

Iodine helps the thyroid gland function correctly and can be found in seafood, iodized salt, and processed foods. Both low and high levels of iodine can result in a lump in the neck called a goiter. This lump is actually the thyroid gland, which has enlarged.

Iron is needed to carry oxygen in the blood and a deficiency of iron can cause anemia. Because oxygen cannot be carried by the blood as effectively when iron is deficient, symptoms of a deficiency include being tired all the time, having no energy, and restlessness. Iron can come from both plant and animal products. The iron from plant products is called nonheme iron. The iron that is found in animal products is called heme iron and is absorbed very well by the body. Sources include meat, fish, poultry, and dark green vegetables.

Manganese is found in fruits, grains, tea, and nuts and helps the bones to form. There are no known affects of low manganese levels, but high levels may affect the brain. Molybdenum is needed to breakdown foods and can be found in leafy green vegetables, legumes, grains, and nuts. Low levels of molybdenum are not known to cause any side effects, but high levels can interfere with the absorption of copper. Selenium is a mineral antioxidant, is involved in the functioning of the thyroid, and is required to breakdown fat. Selenium can be found in fruits and vegetables that are grown in soil that contains the mineral as well as organ meats, seafood, and grain products.

Zinc is very important for proper growth and development, and if a deficiency develops, proper growth cannot take place. You can tell if your child is becoming deficient in zinc by looking at their fingernails. White marks on two or more fingernails may indicate a zinc deficiency. However, these marks will appear before deficiency begins to affect growth. In the diet, zinc can be found in fortified cereals, red meat, and some seafood.

Trace Minerals	Recommended Daily Allowance (RDA) or Adequate Intake		Upper Intake Level
Chromium * Adequate Intake not RDA	Children 4-8 years:	15 mcg	
	Males 9-13 years:	25 mcg	
	Females 9-13 years:	21 mcg	
	Males 14-18 years:	35 mcg	
	Females 14-18 years:	24 mcg	
Copper	Children 4-8 years:	440 mcg	3,000 mcg
	Children 9-13 years:	700 mcg	5,000 mcg
	Males 14-18 years:	890 mcg	8,000 mcg
	Females 14-18 years:	890 mcg	8,000 mcg
Fluoride * Adequate Intake not RDA	Children 4-8 years:	1 mg	2.2 mg
	Children 9-13 years:	2 mg	10 mg
	Males 14-18 years:	3 mg	10 mg
	Females 14-18 years:	3 mg	10 mg

Trace Minerals	Recommended Daily Allowance (RDA) or Adequate Intake		Upper Intake Level
Iodine	Children 4-8 years:	90 mcg	300 mcg
	Children 9-13 years:	120 mcg	600 mcg
	Males 14-18 years:	150 mcg	900 mcg
	Females 14-18 years:	150 mcg	900 mcg
Iron	Children 4-8 years:	10 mg	40 mg
	Children 9-13 years:	8 mg	40 mg
	Males 14-18 years:	11 mg	45 mg
	Females 14-18 years:	15 mg	45 mg
Manganese * Adequate Intake not RDA	Children 4-8 years:	1.5 mg	3 mg
	Males 9-13 years:	1.9 mg	6 mg
	Females 9-13 years:	1.6 mg	6 mg
	Males 14-18 years:	2.2 mg	9 mg
	Females 14-18 years:	1.6 mg	9 mg
Molybdenum	Children 4-8 years:	22 mcg	600 mcg
	Children 9-13 years:	34 mcg	1,100 mcg
	Males 14-18 years:	43 mcg	1,700 mcg
	Females 14-18 years:	43 mcg	1,700 mcg
Selenium	Children 4-8 years:	30 mcg	150 mcg
	Children 9-13 years:	40 mcg	280 mcg
	Males 14-18 years:	55 mcg	400 mcg
	Females 14-18 years:	55 mcg	400 mcg
Zinc	Children 4-8 years:	5 mg	12 mg
	Children 9-13 years:	8 mg	23 mg
	Males 14-18 years:	11 mg	34 mg
	Females 14-18 years:	9 mg	34 mg

* Source: Dietary Reference Intakes (DRIs): Recommended Intakes for Individuals, Elements. *Food and Nutrition Board, Institute of Medicine, National Academies.* www. iom.edu

Summary Points

❖ *The body requires vitamins in order to use energy from foods.*

❖ *Deficiencies and toxicities of vitamins and minerals can develop.*

❖ *Use a vitamin supplement that is created for children.*

❖ *Water-soluble vitamins include all of the B vitamins and vitamin C.*

❖ *Fat-soluble vitamins include vitamins A, D, E, & K.*

❖ *Excessive intake of the fat-soluble vitamins is more likely to lead to toxicity than excessive intake of the water-soluble vitamins.*

❖ *The B vitamins are required to break down carbohydrates and proteins, to allow enzymes to work properly in the body, to allow for proper division of cells, and to prevent a certain type of anemia.*

❖ *Vitamin C is an antioxidant in the body and helps protect the body against damage.*

❖ *The fat-soluble vitamins are needed to maintain vision, allow for proper growth, are required for the development of the bones, protect against damage, and help the body to clot the blood.*

❖ *The major minerals are needed in large quantities in the body for a variety of functions including maintaining the balance of fluids in the body.*

❖ *Trace minerals are required in smaller quantities than the major minerals, but still have important functions in the body.*

CHAPTER 7

FOOD LABELS MADE EASY

Before being able to choose and buy healthy foods for your child, you need to be able to read a food label. For fruits and vegetables, it's easy. There are no food labels and all fruits and vegetables can be included in your child's health plan. However, with breads, cereals, crackers and other foods, food labels can appear complicated. I will make it easy and provide you with a list of what you will find on a food label, and why the information is important. An example of a food label is on the following page. I have added numbers to the food label that corresponds to numbers in the descriptions below so that you know which area of the food label I am discussing.

NUTRITION FACTS	
Serving Size: 14 chips (1) Servings Per Bag: About 10 (2)	
Amount Per Serving (3)	
Calories 200	Calories From Fat 120 (4)
	% Daily Value
Total Fat 12g (5)	18%
Saturated Fat 10 g Monounsaturated Fat 2g	
Cholesterol 30mg (6)	10%
Sodium 470 mg (7)	20%
Total Carbohydrate 31 g (8)	10%
Dietary Fiber 0 g Sugar 5 g	
Protein 5 g (9)	
Vitamin A 8 % Vitamin C 12% Calcium 18% Iron 3% (10)	

* Percent Daily Values are based on a 2,000-calorie diet. Your daily values may be higher or lower depending on your calories needs.			
	Calories:	2,000	2,500
Total Fat	Less than	65 g	80 g
Sat Fat	Less than	20 g	25 g
Cholesterol	Less than	300 mg	300 mg
Sodium	Less than	2,400 mg	2,400 mg
Total carbohydrate	300 mg	375 mg	
Dietary Fiber	25 g		
(11)			

Ingredient List: potatoes, salt, vinegar (12)

Serving Size and Number of Servings

The first thing that is listed on a food label is the serving size (1). This is important because all of the information on the rest of the label, including fat content, only refers to the amount in that serving. Using the example food label, you can see that a serving size is 14 chips, if your child ate 28 chips you would take the number of fat grams, calories, and everything else on the label, and double it to know how much your child consumed. This is important because a food may appear to be low in saturated fat, calories, or cholesterol, but when you consider what is actually been consumed, your child may be taking in a large amount from just one food.

The next thing on the food label is the number of servings (2). This is telling you how many servings of a food you should receive from the package that you purchased. If your child eats more than one serving, the package will not last as long. You can also use this information to determine how much of each nutrient your child has consumed. For example, the food label states that a serving is 14 chips and that there are approximately 10 servings per bag. If you child consumed half the bag at one sitting, you would multiply the nutrient information by 5 to determine how much they consumed. If they ate the whole bag, you would multiply by 10.

Amount per Serving

After information about servings on a food label is an area called "Amount per Serving" (3). This tells you how much fat, carbohydrate, cholesterol, sodium and protein is contained in the food based on a serving size. On the food label example, this information would be provided based on consuming 14 chips.

Calories and Calories from Fat

The amount of calories on a food label tells you how much energy the body can receive from consuming the food (4). The "Calories from Fat" section of the food label tells you how much energy is received from the fat contained in the food. The body obtains more energy (or calories) from fat than an equal amount of carbohydrate or protein. No more than 30% of your child's daily calorie intake should come from fat.

Fat

The food label will tell you how much total fat, saturated fat, monounsaturated fat, polyunsaturated fat, and trans fat (5) are in a serving. Trans fats were added as a requirement to food labels as of 2006. Saturated and trans fats are the ones that should be limited in your child's diet. Monounsaturated and polyunsaturated fats are better for your child.

Cholesterol

Food labels will also list the amount of cholesterol contained within a food. As you can see on the example food label, a serving of 14 chips provides 30 mg of cholesterol (6). Adequate amounts of cholesterol are actually very important for the cells of the body to function. Your child needs adequate amounts of cholesterol to grow and develop properly. Cholesterol only becomes dangerous when we have high amounts in our blood because it can deposit along artery walls leading to plaque formation. So, while excessive amounts of cholesterol should be avoided, cholesterol should never be eliminated from your child's diet.

Sodium

The sodium content represents the amount of salt that is in a food (7). Some foods can be higher in sodium than you would think. If food manufacturers remove chloride from sodium chloride, the food does not taste salty. However, if you look at the food label, the food might be high in salt. So, you cannot judge the sodium content of a food based on taste, you must look at the food label. Salt is also used as a preservative to keep foods from going bad. When salt intake is high, the body holds onto water, which can increase the blood pressure.

Total Carbohydrates

The total amount of carbohydrates, including dietary fiber and sugar, must be included on a food label (8). Approximately 60% of your child's daily energy intake should come from carbohydrates, especially whole grains. You should avoid foods that have a high amount of sugar and encourage foods that have a high amount of dietary fiber. Typically, foods that are high in sugar provide what are called "empty calories." In other words, your child receives energy (calories) from consuming the food, but little (if any) other nutrients such as vitamins, minerals, or fiber. "Empty calorie" foods include candy, soda, and other junk foods. You may have heard of a newer term called "Net Carbs," this is a term that came out of the low carbohydrate diet craze. It is a term used by food manufacturers only and is not one assigned by the Food and Drug Administration. To determine the amount of net carbs, manufacturers subtract the amount of fiber and sugar alcohols from the number of total carbohydrates. However, all of these forms of carbohydrates have the potential to raise blood sugar levels, so the term "net carb" is not a beneficial one.

Protein

The number of grams of protein in a serving of food will also be listed on a food label (9). Approximately 10% to 20% of a child's daily energy intake should come from protein. Protein is very important to build the muscles of the body and is essential to proper growth in your child. Typically, foods that come from animals are high in protein, such as meat, poultry, fish, eggs, and milk products.

Vitamins and Minerals

Next is the list of vitamins and minerals. The label will tell you the percentage of the Recommended Daily Allowance that a serving size of a food provides for certain vitamins and minerals (10). While some food labels list all vitamins and minerals contained in the food, the only ones required to be on a label are vitamin C, vitamin A, iron, and calcium. All four of these nutrients are required for the proper growth and development of your child.

2,000 and 2,500 Calorie Diets

Most food labels will list the amount of fat, cholesterol, sodium, and total carbohydrate that are required for a 2,000 and 2,500 calorie diet (11). The problem with this is that depending upon the age of your child, 2,000 calories per day may be too much. See chapter 3 for the specific amount of servings required for your child based on age.

Ingredients

On the bottom of a nutrition label, you will find the list of ingredients (12). Whatever is listed first is contained in the product the most. For example, if the ingredient list states that a product contains potatoes, salt, and vinegar, potatoes would be found the most and vinegar the least in the product. You should avoid buying products that have sugar listed as the first or second ingredient. If you do buy these products, your child's consumption of them should be limited.

Other Label Items

You may also see statements on a label that characterize the quality of a nutrient in a food. For example, fat-free, cholesterol-free, or low-calorie are statements you have probably seen on foods before. The Food and Drug Administration regulates a manufacturer's right to claim that a food is free of or low in calories, fat, cholesterol, sodium, or sugar. The product must meet certain guidelines to use those terms. However, there are other terms that manufacturers often place on the front of a product to attract consumers. These catch phrases tend to change with time depending upon the mindset that is popular at that moment. I already gave you one example, which is "net carbs," but another big one is "all-natural." A potato, even if it is deep-fried in oil with a high amount of saturated fat, is all-natural. It grew in the ground, didn't it? So, it is all-natural. Don't be fooled by these marketing schemes. You now know how to read a food label to make sure you are buying a food that is healthy for you and your child.

Involving Kids

You will not always be there when your child is making decisions about what foods to buy or eat. Because of that, it is incredibly important that they learn how to read a food label as well. If you have children who are old enough to read, you can make a game out of reading food labels while you are in the grocery store. You can make the game "who can find the food with the least amount of sodium or saturated fat," or "who can find the food with the most calcium or fiber." If you have two children they can play the game with each other, if not you and your child can play the game together. Not only will this teach your child how to read a food label, but also keeps your child occupied while shopping so they are not distracted by high fat and high sugar foods. For older children, you can have them compare two different brands of the same type of food and see if they can determine which one is healthier.

Vitamin Supplement Labels

There are also labels on the side of vitamin supplement bottles. These labels are different from what you would see on a food product. On a vitamin supplement label, there will be a list of all of the vitamins and mineral contained in the product, the number of micrograms, milligrams, or grams of each vitamin and mineral, and the percentage of the Recommended Daily Allowance (RDA) that is met by consuming the vitamins. Make sure you pay attention to the serving size. If it says, "Serving Size: 2 tablets," then you must consume two tablets to receive what is listed on the vitamin supplement label.

When choosing a vitamin supplement for your child, choose one that has no more than 100% of the RDA for any of the vitamins or minerals contained in the product. If you choose a product that has 200 or 300 times the RDA, the toxicity symptoms that were discussed in the vitamins and minerals chapter may develop. Some vitamin supplements also contain herbs. Herbs may affect children differently than they do adults, so again, make sure you choose a vitamin supplement that is specifically made for children. If you have Internet access, look up information about the vitamin supplement before deciding on a particular brand. There are independent companies that analyze vitamin supplements to make sure they contain what the label says the product contains and analyze for unwanted products such as lead.

Summary Points

❖ *Knowing the serving size of a food is important because all information on a food label is only the amount present in a single serving.*

❖ *The number of servings refers to approximately how many servings you should receive from a package.*

❖ *The "Amount per Serving" tells you how much fat, carbohydrate, cholesterol, sodium and protein are contained in a food based on the serving size.*

❖ *The number of calories tells you how much energy the body will receive from a food.*

❖ *The "Calories from Fat" will tell you how many of the calories in a food come from fat.*

❖ *The label will list the amount of total fat, saturated fat, monounsaturated fat, polyunsaturated fat, and trans fats that are in one serving.*

❖ *The amount of cholesterol in a serving will be listed on the label. Foods that are high in cholesterol should be avoided.*

❖ *The amount of sodium present in a serving will be listed. Foods with high sodium content should be avoided.*

❖ *The amount of carbohydrates including dietary fiber and sugar will be listed.*

❖ *The amount of protein will be listed and should represent 10% to 20% of a child's daily energy intake.*

❖ *The percentage of the Recommended Daily Allowance for vitamin C, vitamin A, iron, and calcium will be listed. Occasionally products will list all vitamins and minerals.*

❖ *The amount of fat, cholesterol, sodium, and total carbohydrate required for a 2,000 and 2,500 calorie diet will be listed.*

❖ *Ingredients will be listed on the food label based on the amount of the ingredient that is in the food with those present in the highest amounts listed first.*

❖ *Statements on a food label about the quality of a nutrient are often regulated by the Food and Drug Administration.*

- ❖ *It is important to teach children how to read a food label.*
- ❖ *Vitamin supplement labels should be read, and products with more than 100% of the RDA for any vitamin or mineral should be avoided.*

CHAPTER 8

BEATING EMOTIONAL EATING

There are many causes of obesity. Genetics, medications, and eating patterns can all influence an individual's weight. However, there is also an emotional aspect that influences some people when they are deciding what to eat and how much to eat. Many adults turn to food for comfort when they are upset or under stress, and children are no different. For adults stress is usually caused by work, but for kids stress can come from school or home. Children may turn to food because they did poorly on a test, had trouble with a friend, are being picked on at school, or are upset about something going on at home. They may use food as a method to cope with their stress.

Think about the first time someone tried to calm your child down by using food. Odds are one of the first places this happened was your child's health care provider's office. Many offer lollipops as a reward for good behavior or to calm your child down after they have received a shot. Some parents also use food as a reward. Have you ever said to your child: "If you're good, I will give you a cookie"? You can substitute the word "cookie" with whatever type of food you offered; maybe it was candy or fast food. Everyone has probably done that at some time, but using food as a reward can be the beginning of a child's emotional relationship with food. The child learns to turn to food when they are feeling unhappy, stressed, or depressed because in the past, food made them feel better.

Coping mechanisms are methods individual's use to cope with stress; some are healthy and some are not. Turning to food is an unhealthy way to cope. So how do you teach your child new coping mechanisms? Remember, you are your child's role model. Think about how you cope with stress. Do you turn to food? Do you bottle things up inside until you reach a boiling point? Do you take out your frustrations from work on those at home? All of these are common unhealthy coping mechanisms. By learning new ways to cope with stress yourself, you can also teach your child how to better deal with problems. The following are some examples of healthy coping mechanisms you and your child can use:

- ❖ Go for a walk
- ❖ Listen to music
- ❖ Write down feelings
- ❖ Talk to family and friends about problems
- ❖ Participate in exercise, sports, or yoga
- ❖ Play a musical instrument
- ❖ Get adequate rest and sleep
- ❖ Think positive self-thoughts (more about this later)

To discourage the use of food as a reward, ask your child's health care provider if they will give your child something other than candy (like a sticker) at the end of their visit. Most health care providers will be more than willing to change, especially when asked by a parent. If you have used food in the past as a reward, you should also think of something else to offer your child. Spending an hour or a day in the park or at the beach can be just as much fun for your child as receiving candy as a reward.

Is Your Child an Emotional Eater?

Not all children are emotional eaters, so it is important to determine if your child is eating in response to stress. If your child is old enough, usually over 11 years, you can have them complete the Emotion Log for 2 weeks. For younger children (6-10 years old), you can ask them how they feel and fill out the form for them. After the two-week period, take the forms and look them over. If your child says they felt a negative emotion before eating a food followed by a positive emotion while eating or after eating a food, they are probably an emotional eater. Some kids will say they felt guilt, shame, or disappointment after eating a food, which is a strong sign of emotional eating. Children sometimes have difficulty placing a name to an emotion, so having a list of emotions can help them identify what they are feeling. If your child is an emotional eater, then they need to be taught the different ways to cope with stress that were mentioned previously.

Emotion Log			
Date:_____			

Before I ate _____, I felt _____.
While I was eating _____, I felt _____.
After eating _____, I felt _____.

Before I ate _____, I felt _____.
While I was eating _____, I felt_____.
After eating _____, I felt _____.

Before I ate _____, I felt _____.
While I was eating _____, I felt _____.
After eating _____, I felt _____.

Before I ate _____, I felt _____.
While I was eating _____, I felt _____.
After eating _____, I felt _____.

Before I ate _____, I felt _____.
While I was eating _____, I felt _____.
After eating _____, I felt _____.

LIST OF EMOTIONS

Angry	Anxious	Bored	Calm
Comforted	Depressed	Disappointed	Fearful
Guilty	Happy	Hopeful	Lonely
Nervous	Pain	Proud	Remorse
Sad	Shame	Unhappy	Worry

You Can Do It!

Think of a time in your life when you truly wanted to accomplish something. Who did you turn to for support? More than likely it was a family member, the constants in out lives. Now imagine what it would be like to try to accomplish something with no support from family. It would be very difficult, wouldn't it?

Your child needs the support of your entire family while changing their lifestyle to follow this health plan. As I said in the beginning of this book, you are a role model to your child. If you are living a very unhealthy lifestyle, the odds of this plan being effective for your child are slim if you continue to live that lifestyle. But, if you think about the long term benefits following this plan will have for your child, it is worth it. Think of how much you have sacrificed for your child to give them a good life. Making this lifestyle change will not be a sacrifice; it will be beneficial for the whole family.

Feeling Good

Self-esteem involves your child's feelings about themselves and their self-worth. Family members including siblings, kids at school, and the media can affect self-esteem. If there are siblings in the family, it will be extremely helpful to forbid jokes and comments about weight, not only about overweight but also underweight. Of course, you cannot be with your children every second of every day, but if you hear these comments, put a stop to them. The self-esteem of your child will increase if they know that you will not tolerate these comments and they will believe that you support them.

Negative comments about weight may also come from other kids at school, and can make children very upset. Unfortunately, no matter what someone's weight, height, or other attributes, there will always be people with negative things to say. It can be helpful to talk with teachers or parents about comments that are being made by other children. With a strong support system at home and healthy coping mechanisms, children can learn to ignore negative comments from other people. However, when negative comments start coming from the child about themselves, this mindset can be damaging to their sense of self-worth. Teaching your child to have positive self-thoughts can be very helpful.

Mind over Matter

The mind is more powerful than most people give it credit for. When your child is constantly saying negative comments to themselves (whether they are vocalized or not), their self-esteem begins to decline. You can help train your child to think positively about themselves and their abilities. Write the following on a piece of paper and have your child fill it out everyday:

- ❖ I feel good when I _____.
- ❖ I am good at _____.
- ❖ Three good things about myself are _____.

If you have a young child, you can ask them to complete the sentence as you read it aloud. It may be difficult for your child to complete this at first. They may even get frustrated and not want to complete the sentences. If that is the case, they have been thinking about themselves negatively for so long that is has become very hard for them to think of anything positive. You can help your child for the first week or two (especially with the "three good things" about themselves). However, to create changes in their self-thoughts, they need to begin thinking of these positive attributes on their own.

If you find that your child is always focusing on appearance, encourage them to think about good things they did for other people, how they made other people feel, how they are doing in school, or other abilities. It is important for children to understand that it is not what they look like that makes them a good person. Refocusing the child from appearances to personality and behavior aids in reinforcing the belief that being a good person is what is most important.

The Weight and Food Message

Your child is bombarded with messages about food and weight all day long from the media. Magazines, TV commercials, the news, the radio, and even billboards on the streets send messages to your child about what they should eat and what they should look like. Unfortunately, these forms of media often lead children to develop unrealistic expectations about what they should look like and promote foods that are usually bad for your child's health.

If you have young children, have you sat down to watch cartoons with your child lately? Nearly every commercial is trying to sell your child something, or more specifically, make them want something to the point that they will beg you for it. To encourage your child to want a food, they often attach a cartoon character to the product. When you get to the grocery store, the products that have been advertised to your kids on television are placed at your child's eye level so that the product catches their attention.

To avoid these messages from the media, your child would have to walk around with earplugs and a blindfold. Obviously, that is not an option. So, what can you do to help control how these messages affect your child? Here are some suggestions:

Grocery shopping:

❖ If possible, have someone baby-sit your child while you go food shopping.

❖ If you bring your child to the grocery store with you, use the food label game to distract your child.

❖ You can also distract your child by using a treasure hunt in the grocery store. Before heading out to the store, write a list of some of the foods that you want to purchase. As you walk up and down the isles, your child will be busy looking for the products and hopefully will not become overly obsessed with the objects that he/she has seen in advertising.

Watching TV:

❖ For young children that are heavily influenced by television ads, consider recording the shows that your child likes and fast forward through the commercials.

❖ For older children, have them count the number of commercials during one show that are for food. Have them keep track of how many of the food commercials are for fast food. Then, have them keep track of how many of the commercials are for weight loss products or programs. Discuss with your child how commercials are created to sell a product and often do not mention the bad aspects of a food, product, or program.

❖ Talk to your child about how he or she is targeted by television ads. For example, during a show whose audience is typically young girls, there are usually commercials that talk about appearance (like blemishes). Often these ads try to make your child have a lower self-esteem about a particular feature and want to convince your child that their product will improve a specific area. Talk to your child about food commercials and how they use people that are the same age as those watching the show to convince them to purchase a particular food, which is almost always an unhealthy food.

Listening to the radio:

❖ You can use the same method of counting commercials and discussion mentioned under "watching TV".

❖ If you have a child who is heavily influenced by radio commercials, consider satellite radio, which does not have commercials.

Reading magazines:

❖ Usually magazine advertisers focus more on appearance and weight rather than food.

❖ You can discuss the use of airbrushing with your child. Tell them that pictures of people are often airbrushed to remove blemishes on the skin or to make a person appear thinner. Knowing that models in pictures are not as flawless as they may appear can be helpful to your child.

❖ Your children read and hear about young celebrities and see these celebrities making wrong choices and often ending up in drug or alcohol rehabilitation. Use this as an opportunity to teach your child that no one can be perfect and that what is important is being healthy and happy. Talk about how the media influences these young celebrities to desire perfection, and when they cannot reach perfection, they begin making wrong choices.

Real Life Lesson

When I was a nurse practitioner student, I was taking care of a 13-year-old boy that I will refer to as John. At the age of 13, John was 210 pounds and already had high cholesterol levels. Despite the fact that John had been inactive for the past 3 years, he wanted me to sign a physical form saying that he could play football in school. Because of his cholesterol levels and long-term inactivity, I refused. Yes, he needed exercise, but going from no activity to football was too dramatic of a change, and I was afraid his heart couldn't handle it, even at 13. He was upset with me at first, but after explaining my concerns, he understood.

We spoke for a while about his eating and activity patterns. He told me that he was fine until dinner, but that he would eat snack foods all night long in front of the television until he went to bed. I asked John if he ate so much at night because he was hungry or because he was bored. He couldn't answer the question. Thankfully, we had four months before the physical form had to be turned in, so John and I made a deal. I gave him a list of things to do, and if his cholesterol levels were better, I would reconsider. He really wanted to play football, so that was plenty of motivation. I gave John the following list:

Snacks:
1. *Ask your parents to purchase healthier snacks like baked chips, pretzels, fruits, or vegetables.*
2. *Before you eat a snack, ask yourself: "Am I hungry?" If the answer is "no," don't eat a snack.*
3. *If you are hungry while watching television and want a snack, go to a room like the kitchen or dining room where you can't see the television and eat your snack there.*

Activity:
1. *Go for a 15-minute walk every day for two weeks, increasing the pace each day.*

2. *After two weeks, do 30 minutes of any type of activity for another two weeks.*

3. *In one-week intervals, increase the amount of activity to 45-minutes, then at least 60-minutes.*

Emotional Eating Log

1. *Complete the emotional eating log for two weeks.*

I also gave John a pedometer that would track the number of steps he took each day. I told him to write down the number of steps he had walked at the end of the day. I asked him to try to increase the number of steps he took every day.

Two weeks later, I called John to discuss the emotional eating log. He said he now had an answer to my question, "I was eating because I was bored." He said that he used to eat a whole bag of potato chips in two nights and now the bag is lasting a whole week, and they were baked potato chips. He said that walking away from the television to eat was helping because he didn't want to miss his shows so he spent less time eating. He was also in front of the television less because of the activity schedule I had given him.

I checked in on his progress several time over the next couple of months and he always said he was doing better and better. Four months went by quickly and John came to see me. He walked through the door with a big smile on his face and waving his physical form. When I weighed him, he had lost 20 pounds and his cholesterol levels were back into normal ranges. I happily signed the physical form and he did quite well in his first year of high school football.

Summary Points

❖ *Children may turn to food as a method of coping with stress.*

❖ *Adopt healthy coping mechanisms and teach these strategies to your child.*

❖ *Do not use food as a reward.*

❖ *Determine if your child is an emotional eater.*

❖ *Foster a supportive family environment.*

❖ *Self-esteem may be affected by comments from siblings and/or class-mates.*

❖ *Teach your child to think positive self-thoughts.*

❖ *Consider the influence of media over your child's thoughts about food and weight.*

CHAPTER 9

MOVING AND GROOVING TO BETTER HEALTH

Those who are physically inactive lead what is called a sedentary lifestyle. Being inactive can lead to many health problems. The human body is made to move. If you were stuck in one position, unable to move, your body would slowly begin to deteriorate. Despite the fact that most of us were born with the ability to move and exercise, many find physical activity to be a chore. But, activity is essential to good health and your child cannot become truly healthy unless physical activity becomes part of their life. There are many benefits to physical activity, including the following:

❖ Exercise is important for the muscles because it makes them stronger and allows the body to perform movement better.
❖ Exercise helps increase the density and strength of the bones.
❖ With physical activity, the brain receives more oxygen so it can function better and can help improve concentration and academic performance.
❖ Exercise is important for increasing the functioning of the heart and the lungs.
❖ Exercise increases self-esteem.
❖ Regular physical activity decreases the risk of coronary heart disease, stroke, type II diabetes, and high blood pressure (CDC, 2006).

Coronary heart disease, stroke, type II diabetes, and high blood pressure may sound like problems only adults encounter; however, children are experiencing these problems at an alarming rate. Type II diabetes used to be known as adult onset diabetes, but this is changing due to the number of children being diagnosed with the condition. Obesity and type II diabetes are closely related. When people are diagnosed with type II diabetes in adulthood, it can result in problems with the kidneys, eyes, and circulatory system. When children are diagnosed with the condition, it is even more frightening because all of these problems can develop at a much earlier age. Thankfully, type II diabetes and obesity can be controlled with proper diet and exercise.

Activity Classes

Physical activities are typically classified as either aerobic or anaerobic. Aerobic activities use the major muscle groups of the body, involve the use of oxygen, elevate the heart rate, and are sustained for an extended period of time. This type of activity is very beneficial to the cardiac, vascular, and respiratory body systems. Anaerobic activity involves short bursts of intense exercise that help to increase muscle mass. Both types of activities are beneficial to your child, and both should be included in their daily activity patterns. Following is a list of some aerobic and anaerobic activities.

AEROBIC ACTIVITIES

- ❖ Bicycling
- ❖ Canoeing
- ❖ Dancing
- ❖ Jogging
- ❖ Jumping rope
- ❖ Hiking
- ❖ Hockey
- ❖ Kayaking
- ❖ Marching band
- ❖ Rollerblading
- ❖ Rowing
- ❖ Running
- ❖ Skating
- ❖ Skiing
- ❖ Swimming
- ❖ Tennis
- ❖ Walking
- ❖ Walking the dog

ANAEROBIC ACTIVITIES

- ❖ Baseball
- ❖ Basketball
- ❖ Bowling
- ❖ Boxing
- ❖ Fishing
- ❖ Football
- ❖ Golf
- ❖ Gymnastics
- ❖ Handball
- ❖ Skateboarding
- ❖ Soccer
- ❖ Softball
- ❖ Sprinting
- ❖ Stretching
- ❖ Tai Chi
- ❖ Weightlifting
- ❖ Wrestling
- ❖ Yoga

Aerobic and anaerobic activities can even be included when you are having your child do household chores. Aerobic activities include mowing the lawn, raking leaves, shoveling snow, sweeping, and vacuuming. Anaerobic activities include washing windows, dusting, or doing the laundry.

Sixty is the Key

It is recommended that children and adolescents should participate in at least 60 minutes of moderate intensity activities on a daily basis (Strong et al., 2005). However, if your child has been leading a sedentary lifestyle, in other words they have been physically inactive; going directly to 60 minutes might be difficult for them. A slow increase in activity to increase the strength of the heart and muscles will be more beneficial for your child. Start with 15 minutes of activity everyday for 2 weeks. After the initial two weeks, increase the activity to 30 minutes for another two weeks. After the first month, increase physical activity time to 45 and 60 minutes in one-week intervals. In other words:

- ❖ At the start of the Health Plan for Overweight Children: 2 weeks of 15 minutes of activity.
- ❖ Two weeks of 30 minutes of activity.
- ❖ One week of 45 minutes of activity.

❖ One week later and anytime after the 1st 5 weeks: 60 minutes of activity.

If your child has been physically active before beginning the Health Plan for Overweight Children, increase the amount of physical activity they participate in by 15 minutes per week until you reach a minimum of 60 minutes of activity.

Caution: Children who are beginning to engage in physical activity should see a health care provider and have a physical exam before becoming active.

No More Excuses

When some people hear the words "physical activity," they automatically think of football, basketball, baseball, soccer, and other team sports. It becomes easy to say, "My child just does not like those types of activities." There are many ways to increase activity that do not involve organized sports. There are ways to encourage physical activity among children who like music, art, and even video games.

For the child that likes music:

❖ If your child is old enough, encourage them to join a marching band.
❖ If they play an instrument, have them dance or walk as they play.
❖ Encourage them to join a dancing class.
❖ Encourage them to dance to music at home.
❖ Play a game with your child and see who can come up with the silliest dance moves.

For the child that likes art:

❖ Take a walk in the park with your child to find something that they can draw or paint.
❖ Go for a walk on the beach to find something your child can draw or paint.

For the child that likes video games:

❖ Purchase video games that involve physical activity. There are games that involve moving the feet to images seen on the screen.
❖ If you are purchasing a video game system, consider purchasing a video game system that promotes physical activity among those

playing the games. There are video game systems available where children can choose from golf, tennis, bowling, and many other activity games.

Motivation for Mobilization

Organized sports are great for children. In addition to being physically active, they learn about how to work with others, a skill that will benefit them throughout life. However, participation in these types of activities should be based on your child's desire to be in an organized sport. Pushing your child to play soccer because you missed the opportunity when you were younger will just result in tension between you and your child. Allow your child the opportunity to choose an activity.

It is so important for you as a parent to remember that it is just the participation in the sport that is important, not the outcome of the event. In other words, it does not matter if your child wins or loses, just that they have the team sport experience. Parental focus on the outcome of their child's sporting events has resulted in some rather disturbing displays in our society. Having a parent be arrested and/or jailed for poor or illegal conduct at a child's sporting event is becoming more common. This places an enormous amount of stress on your child and does not teach them the right way to deal with losing or conflict.

Gender roles can become a conflict with some parents when it comes to participation in activities. Does it really matter if you have a son who wants to be in a dance class or in gymnastics or a daughter who wants to play hockey or lacrosse? You need to keep in mind what is really important. Does your child enjoy what they are doing? If the answer is yes, that is all that should matter.

Create and Participate

Your child will love being physically active if it is fun for them. When activity is too structured, it becomes too much like work. Some children will enjoy physical activity videos that are geared toward kids. However, many children become bored due to the repetition. Climbing on a jungle gym, playing tag with other kids in the neighborhood, playing hopscotch, or jumping rope are all different forms of activity that most children enjoy doing. They do not consider these types of activities as exercise, usually they think of it as playtime.

You can encourage creativity in your child by allowing them to develop a game that involves running, jumping, skipping, or any other activity. Let them develop the rules to the game and how it will be played. This allows them to be physically active, but also helps them develop their creativity skills.

Reward System

Parents can motivate their children to engage in physical activity using the same reward system presented in Chapter Two. There are additional rewards charts in Appendix A of this book. As a reminder, the rewards that you choose should not be related to food. You can give your child a star for each 15 minutes of activity in which they participate. When they achieve a certain number of stars, they receive a reward. A great thing to do is to incorporate physical activity into the reward. For the child that enjoys activity, you may include a reward such as renting a paddleboat at a local lake, taking your child to a skateboarding park, or allowing them to take a class at the local community center. For children who enjoy art, the reward could be a new drawing set or pad. For those who like music, you may want to use a local concert or dance as a reward. These are only examples, discover what you child truly enjoys and build rewards around this.

Another idea is to use the amount of physical activity time your child participates in to determine how much TV, non-exercise based video game, or computer (non-homework related) time the child is allowed. For every 15 minutes of activity, they can receive 15 minutes of time to do non-physical activities.

What you see is what you get

Just as you are a role model when it comes to eating habits, you are also a role model for your child when it comes to physical activity. If you are inactive, your child is much more likely to do the same. Participating in physical activity with your child will not only increase the health of both you and your child, but also give you the opportunity to bond.

Risk Reduction

Physical activity benefits your child in many ways. However, there are also safety issues that need to be considered. If proper care is taken, the risk for injury while being physically active can be minimized.

Before engaging in activity, it is important for your child to stretch to prevent injuring the muscles. Organized sport activities should include stretching before practice and events (also know as a warm-up). For young children, you can play a game of Simon Says to encourage stretching. Include movements that stretch the leg, arm, and back muscles. For older children, they may enjoy doing yoga before other activities. Yoga involves movements that will stretch the muscles.

There are several activities where children should wear protective equipment while participating. Children who enjoy bicycling should wear a bike helmet (they are more likely to wear one if you do as well). Many organized sports such as football, soccer, baseball, and hockey use protective equipment. You want to ensure that the equipment is the proper size. Protective equipment that is too big or small may result in injury. If your child enjoys rollerblading or skateboarding, there are kneepads, elbow pads, and helmets that can be worn to prevent injury. No matter how careful you and your child are, injuries may occur. If an injury does develop, make sure you seek medical attention.

It is also important to make sure that your child stays well hydrated during physical activity. Sweat is important because it allows the body to cools itself as it evaporates from the skin. But, when this occurs, the body is losing water and that water loss needs to be replaced. If your child is participating in anaerobic activities that are usually short in duration, water is enough to replace losses. But, with aerobic activities replacing water is not enough; both water and electrolytes need to be replaced. Drinks like Gatorade® or Powerade® are beneficial to replace lost water and electrolytes. Because of caffeine and high sugar content, soda results in a loss of water and should be avoided.

You also need to use caution if the temperature outside is very warm or very cold. Hyperthermia occurs when the body's temperature goes very high, just as if you have a fever. This can occur due to activity that is performed in hot weather. If your child starts to feel dizzy, weak, nauseous, or has cold clammy skin, place them in the shade, put a washcloth in cool water and place it over the forehead or behind the neck, and provide water or juice. If the child becomes disoriented, confused, or combative, seek medical attention. The opposite problem is hypothermia, a low body temperature, which can occur due to activity that is performed in cold weather. Symptoms can progress from shivering and grogginess to unconsciousness, difficulty breathing, and a lack of shivering. For the initial symptoms, you should encourage your child to drink warm fluids, move into a warm dry area, and put on extra layers of clothing. For later symptoms, you should seek medical attention.

Real Life Lessons

Do not underestimate the difference that physical activity can make in a child. I had a nursing student whose son was getting in trouble at school on a regular basis. She was getting fed up with the letters and phone calls that she was receiving from the school. Apparently, to say her son was bouncing off the walls at school was an understatement. She had made plans to see a doctor because she thought her child might have Attention Deficit Hyperactivity Disorder (ADHD).

My student was sharing her frustration with me, so I asked her two questions, what does your son eat in a typical day and how much activity does he get? For breakfast he ate two Poptarts and a chocolate milk drink and for lunch he typically had pizza and soda. But, she always made sure he had a healthy dinner. The school her son attended did not have a physical education (PE) program, so he had no activity during the day. When he got home, he would do his homework, eat dinner, play on the computer, and watch television.

I asked her to put off the doctors appointment for one month. In that month, I asked her to change her son's breakfast to a low sugar cereal, fruit and orange juice. For lunch, I recommended sandwiches with peanut butter, chicken, or turkey; water, tea, or green tea to drink; and a piece of fruit. While there was nothing that could be done immediately about the school PE program, I asked her to set aside one hour after school for her son to be active. Before doing homework, he rode his bike, played basketball with his friends, or walked around the neighborhood.

Within a week, she started noticing differences. Her son was finishing his homework faster and improving his grades on assignments (thanks to more oxygen going to his brain). By the end of the month, the letters and phone calls from the school completely stopped. My student called me and told me she canceled the doctor's appointment and couldn't believe the difference changing his food and activity made.

One week later, she received a phone call from one of his teachers. Her first thought was, "here we go again." This time it was a phone call saying what a difference the teacher had seen in her son. But, guess what the teacher asked her, "what kind of medication has your son been put on?" Isn't that sad! We have become a society that thinks that everything in life needs a pill to be fixed. Yes, it might be easier to use pills, but at what cost? Pills have side effects, interactions, and often unknown adverse side effects. If something can be fixed by changing what you do and what you eat, isn't that actually easier that putting up with all of the potential dangers of a pill? By the way, my student soon wrote a letter to the school board asking for the PE program to be reinstated.

Summary Points

❖ *Physical activity is essential to good health.*

❖ *Your child should participate in both aerobic and anaerobic activities.*

❖ *Slowly increase the amount of physical activity your child participates in by 15-minute intervals to a minimum of 60 minutes.*

❖ *Children who enjoy music, art, and video games can also be active.*

❖ *Participation in organized sports should be based on the child's desire to be involved in a team sport.*

❖ *Allow your child to be creative and make activity fun.*

❖ *Rewards can be helpful in encouraging activity.*

❖ *Be a good role model for activity patterns.*

❖ *Use stretching and protective equipment to prevent injuries in your child.*

❖ *Make sure your child stays well hydrated during activity and closely monitor activity in temperature extremes.*

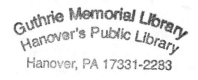

Chapter 10

CHALLENGES OF SINGLE PARENTHOOD AND TWO-PARENT WORKING FAMILIES

Despite the fact that you want what is best for your child and you want your child to be healthy, the challenges of raising a family on your own or having two full-time working parents can be overwhelming. If a child comes home after school and there is no one to supervise food and activity choices, it can be difficult to change a child's behavior pattern. While it may be difficult, it is not impossible.

The first challenge that will be addressed is snacking. Typically, when children come home from school, they are famished and cannot wait until dinnertime to eat something. Use some of the same techniques mentioned in earlier chapters. Leave fruit on the counter where it is visible. Place fruit and vegetables that are in the refrigerator in clear plastic bags so that your child can see them. Leave a note on the refrigerator with a list of healthy snacks that your child can choose from. Limit the amount of junk food in the house as much as possible. If you do have junk food in the house, choose the healthier options like baked potato chips and pretzels.

I have heard health care professionals recommend that parents place a pad lock on the refrigerator when parents are not home. I completely disagree with this thinking. It does not help children learn to regulate their own intake, and I think this is cruel and unreasonable. What if your child really needs something to drink besides water? What do you think this does to a child's self-esteem? The purpose of this plan is to raise self-esteem to modify behavior, not to assist in a decline in self-worth. Please *do not* place padlocks on the refrigerator. If there are healthy foods in the refrigerator, there is no need to lock it up.

Some children have to prepare dinner because parents are working. The problem is that children often want microwavable or fast foods that are high in sodium, high in saturated fat, and provide little nutrition. If you make large meals on the weekend, you can save leftovers in individual portions for your child to eat during the week. Another option is to cook meals each night and your child can reheat the food for dinner the next day. Get your child involved as much as possible. For example, if your child will be eating alone, let him or her pick out dinners for the week (as long as they are healthy). You can place the food in individual sized servings and label them with the days of the week, Monday through Friday. Children may be more likely to eat food if they choose the dinner and know what they are coming home to eat.

Family meals can be more difficult when you are raising a child on your own or have to work until late. Family meals do not have to revolve around dinner. If you work until late, have breakfast together. If you have more than one child, encourage them to eat dinner together at the kitchen or dining room table. On weekends, try to have as many meals together as possible.

While children may have a snack when they first get home from school because they are hungry, they may continue to eat because they are bored. Activity will prevent children from eating more due to boredom. How can you get your child to be active when you are not there to supervise? Find chores around the house that involve activity and that you can tell were performed. Have your child empty the dishwasher, wash dishes, vacuum, or wash counter tops or windows. This not only helps you out, but also keeps your child active. Some parents will say that their child rushes to get the chores done so that they can then sit down and watch television. I say, let them rush. If they run around the house vacuuming and washing the counter tops, they are getting the heart rate elevated and they are physically active. The alternative of not making them do chores will result in more inactivity.

Another option to consider is an after-school activity program. Local community centers and schools often have programs to keep children active when school ends. This may provide your child with something to do until you get home from work. If you have a child who loves to play video games, choose games or video game systems that will keep them active. If you have tried everything and you still have a child who sits and watches television for hours when no one is home, consider blocking the channels that have their favorite shows until a later time of the day.

If your child has a lot of homework to do, have them work on it while you are not at home. When you do get home from work, you can participate in some activity with your child. However, physical activity should not be engaged in within 2 hours of going to sleep. It will be more difficult for your child to fall asleep if they are active before bedtime. If children do not have a lot of time during the week to be physically active, include as much physical activity on the weekends as possible.

Summary Points

- ❖ *Have healthy foods available for after school snacking.*
- ❖ *Have pre-cooked meals available if you are not able to be home for dinner.*
- ❖ *If you are not able to be home for dinner, have a family meal at breakfast.*
- ❖ *Encourage activity while you are away from home by assigning chores.*
- ❖ *Consider after school community center or school programs.*
- ❖ *Include as much physical activity on the weekends as possible.*
- ❖ *Children should not be active within two hours of going to sleep because it will interfere with sleep.*

Chapter 11

DIETARY CHANGES, ACTIVITY CHANGES, and BEST CHOICES

This is the area where many books would provide you with a list of recipes. Whenever I read a book that provides recipes, there's maybe one or two that I would actually use. I think recipe lists are far too restrictive and do not take into account that everyone likes different styles of food. Only you know what your family likes to eat. So, instead I will summarize the diet and activity changes that I made in previous chapters and give you suggestions for the best choices of several categories of foods. You can substitute these healthier options in the recipes you and your family enjoy.

Remember, begin by changing the foods your child currently consumes with healthier options. Then decrease portion sizes until you reach the appropriate number of servings for your child's age. The rate at which you make these changes will depend on your child. If you have a child who is resistant to changes in their diet, progress slowly. For example, begin by replacing meats with healthier options, when your child becomes accustomed to the healthier meat, move on to milk and drinks, then snacks, etc. Another option is to make changes based on meals. For example, make breakfast healthier, and then move on to lunch, dinner, and snacks.

It has taken your child years to develop poor eating habits, and those habits are not going to be corrected overnight. Be patient. With dedication to making better lifestyle choices, improved physical and mental health will result. Along with this improvement in health, your child will begin to attain a weight that will decrease their risk for diseases later in life.

Diet Changes

❖ Replace high-fat beef or pork with lean cuts of beef or pork then skinless turkey and chicken or fish.

❖ Replace ground beef with lean ground beef then lean ground turkey or chicken.

❖ Replace high sodium, high fat lunchmeats with low sodium, low fat lunchmeats.

❖ Replace whole milk with 2%, then 1 %, then nonfat milk.

❖ Replace soda with 100% juice, water, or nonfat milk.

❖ Replace juice "drinks" or "ades" with 100% juice.

❖ Replace fried foods with baked, steamed, boiled, or broiled foods.

❖ Replace coconut oil, palm oil, palm kernel oil, and cocoa butter with safflower, sesame, canola, and olive oils.

❖ Replace salt with herbs and spices.

❖ Replace white breads, rolls, bagels, and pasta with multigrain or whole-wheat breads, rolls, bagels, and pasta.

❖ Replace white flour with whole-wheat flour.

❖ Replace white rice with brown rice.

❖ Replace ice cream with low fat frozen yogurt then fat free frozen yogurt or sherbet.

❖ Replace cookies, candy, and other junk foods with smoothies, fruits, vegetables, or trail mix.

❖ Replace canned fruit in heavy syrup with fruit in light syrup then fruit packed in juice or water.

❖ Replace high fat cheeses with low fat cheeses.

❖ Replace potato chips with baked chips or pretzels.

❖ Replace fast food with home cooked meals.

Activity Changes

❖ 1st 2 weeks: 15 minutes of activity per day.

❖ 2nd 2 weeks: 30 minutes of activity per day.

❖ 5th week: 45 minutes of activity per day.

❖ 6th week and on: at least 60 minutes of activity per day.

Best Choices

When choosing grains, you want to pick those that provide fiber and nutrients and are low in sodium and added sugars. There are healthy options available when choosing breads, rolls, bagels, pasta, rice, flour, cereals, crackers, and other grains.

Breads

- ❖ Cracked wheat
- ❖ Multigrain or mixed grain breads
- ❖ Oat bran
- ❖ Pumpernickel
- ❖ Rye
- ❖ Whole grain waffles or pancakes
- ❖ Whole wheat breads
- ❖ Whole wheat or multigrain English muffins
- ❖ Whole wheat pitas

Rolls and Bagels

- ❖ Multigrain or mixed grain
- ❖ Oat bran
- ❖ Whole wheat

Pasta

- ❖ Multigrain pasta
- ❖ Whole wheat pasta
- ❖ Vegetable pasta

Rice

- ❖ Brown rice
- ❖ Long grain rice
- ❖ Wild Rice

Flour

- ❖ Dark rye
- ❖ Enriched semolina
- ❖ Whole wheat

Cereals

- ❖ Cold:

- o Bran flakes
- o Corn flakes
- o Crisp rice
- o Puffed rice
- o Puffed wheat
- o Shredded wheat
- o Wheat bran
- ❖ Hot:
  - o Cream of rice
  - o Cream of wheat
  - o Farina
  - o Grits
  - o Maypo

Crackers

- ❖ Graham
- ❖ Melba
- ❖ Rye crisps
- ❖ Low sodium saltines

Other grains

- ❖ Barley
- ❖ Bulgur
- ❖ Couscous
- ❖ Cracked wheat
- ❖ Millet
- ❖ Oat bran

Lean meat, poultry, and fish products that are low in saturated fat and low in sodium are the best choice for your child. You can choose healthier options when shopping for beef, pork, chicken, turkey, and fish.

Beef

- ❖ Broiled beef rib
- ❖ Grilled beef chuck
- ❖ Lean beef eye of round (roasted)
- ❖ Lean beef flank
- ❖ Lean beef round
- ❖ Lean round eye

- ❖ Lean top sirloin steak
- ❖ Roasted beef tip round
- ❖ Roasted beef top sirloin
- ❖ 95% Lean ground beef

Pork

- ❖ Extra lean, low sodium ham
- ❖ Lean broiled pork loin
- ❖ Lean center loin chop
- ❖ Lean whole loin chop

Chicken

- ❖ Chicken breast without skin
- ❖ Light meat chicken roll
- ❖ Light meat drumstick without skin
- ❖ Thigh without skin

Turkey

- ❖ Light meat
- ❖ Light meat roll
- ❖ Roasted skinless turkey breast

Fish

- ❖ Cod
- ❖ Grouper
- ❖ Halibut
- ❖ Pollock
- ❖ Snapper
- ❖ Water packed tuna

Dairy products provide an easy way to decrease the amount of saturated fat that is in your child's diet while increasing the amount of calcium your child consumes. There are low and no fat options for cheese, milk, yogurt, and butter.

Cheese

- ❖ American cheese slices
- ❖ Fat free American or cheddar
- ❖ Fat free parmesan

❖ Feta cheese
❖ Low fat cheddar
❖ Low fat cream cheese
❖ Low fat (1%) or nonfat cottage cheese
❖ Nonfat or part skim mozzarella
❖ Romano cheese

Milk

❖ 1% milk
❖ Canned-evaporated skim milk
❖ Dried-instant nonfat milk
❖ Skim milk

Yogurt

❖ Fat free yogurt
❖ Low fat yogurt

Butter

❖ Whipped butter

Chapter 3 provides a list of fruits and vegetables, and all fruits and vegetables can be a part of your child's health plan. You can choose healthier options for items like juice, salad dressing, and desserts. When planning your child's diet, include dessert foods sparingly.

Juice

❖ 100% apple juice
❖ 100% cranberry juice
❖ 100% grape juice
❖ 100% grapefruit juice
❖ 100% orange juice
❖ 100% pineapple juice
❖ 100% prune juice

Salad Dressings

❖ Low calorie Italian
❖ Low calorie French
❖ Low calorie mayonnaise

❖ Low calorie ranch
❖ Low calorie thousand island

Desserts

❖ Air popped popcorn
❖ Angel food cake
❖ Baked potato chips
❖ Low fat or fat free frozen yogurt
❖ Pretzels
❖ Pudding prepared with skim milk

Chapter 12

LET THE BATTLE AGAINST OBESITY BEGIN

By reading this book, you have already taken an important step in helping your child become healthier. The next step is to start making changes in your child's eating and activity patterns. Set both short-term and long-term goals so that you and your child can feel like you are successfully following the plan.

Set backs are a part of life, and they do not indicate failure. If after successfully achieving one aspect of the health plan, your child goes back to old lifestyle habits, just start with the changes again. Every day is a new day to make healthier choices.

By following the health plan, your child will have a decrease in their risk for health problems associated with being overweight. Children with healthier hearts, bodies, and minds are happier, calmer, and perform better in school. I would be very happy to never again see a child with heart disease or type II diabetes. But, I can't be there to make sure that every child eats well and exercises. That is where you come in. You are a soldier in the war against childhood obesity and obesity related diseases. Victory comes with your hard work, diligence, and dedication as you influence your child's health for the rest of their life. This plan will not always be easy, but when you look into your child's eyes as you say goodnight, you know the hard work is worth it.

APPENDIX A
Extra Health Plan Reward Sheets

Health Plan Rewards

Reward Goal: _____

Number of Stars Needed: _____

☆	☆	☆	☆	☆	☆	☆	☆	☆	☆
☆	☆	☆	☆	☆	☆	☆	☆	☆	☆
☆	☆	☆	☆	☆	☆	☆	☆	☆	☆
☆	☆	☆	☆	☆	☆	☆	☆	☆	☆
☆	☆	☆	☆	☆	☆	☆	☆	☆	☆
☆	☆	☆	☆	☆	☆	☆	☆	☆	☆
☆	☆	☆	☆	☆	☆	☆	☆	☆	☆

Health Plan Rewards

Reward Goal: _____

Number of Stars Needed: _____

☆	☆	☆	☆	☆	☆	☆	☆	☆	☆
☆	☆	☆	☆	☆	☆	☆	☆	☆	☆
☆	☆	☆	☆	☆	☆	☆	☆	☆	☆
☆	☆	☆	☆	☆	☆	☆	☆	☆	☆
☆	☆	☆	☆	☆	☆	☆	☆	☆	☆
☆	☆	☆	☆	☆	☆	☆	☆	☆	☆
☆	☆	☆	☆	☆	☆	☆	☆	☆	☆

Health Plan Rewards

Reward Goal: _____

Number of Stars Needed: _____

☆	☆	☆	☆	☆	☆	☆	☆	☆	☆
☆	☆	☆	☆	☆	☆	☆	☆	☆	☆
☆	☆	☆	☆	☆	☆	☆	☆	☆	☆
☆	☆	☆	☆	☆	☆	☆	☆	☆	☆
☆	☆	☆	☆	☆	☆	☆	☆	☆	☆
☆	☆	☆	☆	☆	☆	☆	☆	☆	☆
☆	☆	☆	☆	☆	☆	☆	☆	☆	☆

Health Plan Rewards

Reward Goal: _____

Number of Stars Needed: _____

☆	☆	☆	☆	☆	☆	☆	☆	☆	☆
☆	☆	☆	☆	☆	☆	☆	☆	☆	☆
☆	☆	☆	☆	☆	☆	☆	☆	☆	☆
☆	☆	☆	☆	☆	☆	☆	☆	☆	☆
☆	☆	☆	☆	☆	☆	☆	☆	☆	☆
☆	☆	☆	☆	☆	☆	☆	☆	☆	☆
☆	☆	☆	☆	☆	☆	☆	☆	☆	☆

APPENDIX B
Extra Emotional Eating Logs

Emotion Log

Date:_____

Before I ate _____, I felt _____.

While I was eating _____, I felt _____.

After eating _____, I felt _____.

Before I ate _____, I felt _____.

While I was eating _____, I felt _____.

After eating _____, I felt _____.

Before I ate _____, I felt _____.

While I was eating _____, I felt _____.

After eating _____, I felt _____.

Before I ate _____, I felt _____.

While I was eating _____, I felt _____.

After eating _____, I felt _____.

Before I ate _____, I felt _____.

While I was eating _____, I felt _____.

After eating _____, I felt _____.

LIST OF EMOTIONS

Angry	Anxious	Bored	Calm
Comforted	Depressed	Disappointed	Fearful
Guilty	Happy	Hopeful	Lonely
Nervous	Pain	Proud	Remorse
Sad	Shame	Unhappy	Worry

Emotion Log

Date:_____

Before I ate _____, I felt _____.

While I was eating _____, I felt _____.

After eating _____, I felt _____.

Before I ate _____, I felt _____.

While I was eating _____, I felt _____.

After eating _____, I felt _____.

Before I ate _____, I felt _____.

While I was eating _____, I felt _____.

After eating _____, I felt _____.

Before I ate _____, I felt _____.

While I was eating _____, I felt _____.

After eating _____, I felt _____.

Before I ate _____, I felt _____.

While I was eating _____, I felt _____.

After eating _____, I felt _____.

LIST OF EMOTIONS

Angry	Anxious	Bored	Calm
Comforted	Depressed	Disappointed	Fearful
Guilty	Happy	Hopeful	Lonely
Nervous	Pain	Proud	Remorse
Sad	Shame	Unhappy	Worry

Emotion Log

Date:_____

Before I ate _____, I felt _____.

While I was eating _____, I felt _____.

After eating _____, I felt _____.

Before I ate _____, I felt _____.

While I was eating _____, I felt _____.

After eating _____, I felt _____.

Before I ate _____, I felt _____.

While I was eating _____, I felt _____.

After eating _____, I felt _____.

Before I ate _____, I felt _____.

While I was eating _____, I felt _____.

After eating _____, I felt _____.

Before I ate _____, I felt _____.

While I was eating _____, I felt _____.

After eating _____, I felt _____.

LIST OF EMOTIONS

Angry	Anxious	Bored	Calm
Comforted	Depressed	Disappointed	Fearful
Guilty	Happy	Hopeful	Lonely
Nervous	Pain	Proud	Remorse
Sad	Shame	Unhappy	Worry

Emotion Log

Date:_____

Before I ate _____, I felt _____.

While I was eating _____, I felt _____.

After eating _____, I felt _____.

Before I ate _____, I felt _____.

While I was eating _____, I felt _____.

After eating _____, I felt _____.

Before I ate _____, I felt _____.

While I was eating _____, I felt _____.

After eating _____, I felt _____.

Before I ate _____, I felt _____.

While I was eating _____, I felt _____.

After eating _____, I felt _____.

Before I ate _____, I felt _____.

While I was eating _____, I felt _____.

After eating _____, I felt _____.

LIST OF EMOTIONS

Angry	Anxious	Bored	Calm
Comforted	Depressed	Disappointed	Fearful
Guilty	Happy	Hopeful	Lonely
Nervous	Pain	Proud	Remorse
Sad	Shame	Unhappy	Worry

APPENDIX C

Positive Self-Thought
Work Sheets

❖ I feel good when I _____.

❖ I am good at _____.

❖ Three good things about myself are _____.

- -

❖ I feel good when I _____.

❖ I am good at _____.

❖ Three good things about myself are _____.

- -

❖ I feel good when I _____.

❖ I am good at _____.

❖ Three good things about myself are _____.

- -

❖ I feel good when I _____.

❖ I am good at _____.

❖ Three good things about myself are _____.

- -

❖ I feel good when I _____.

❖ I am good at _____.

❖ Three good things about myself are _____.

❖ I feel good when I _____.

❖ I am good at _____.

❖ Three good things about myself are _____.

- -

❖ I feel good when I _____.

❖ I am good at _____.

❖ Three good things about myself are _____.

- -

❖ I feel good when I _____.

❖ I am good at _____.

❖ Three good things about myself are _____.

- -

❖ I feel good when I _____.

❖ I am good at _____.

❖ Three good things about myself are _____.

- -

❖ I feel good when I _____.

❖ I am good at _____.

❖ Three good things about myself are _____.

Disclaimer

The Health Plan for Overweight Children is not a substitute for medical advice. The reader assumes the responsibility for seeking advice from a health care provider before following this plan. The information and advice presented may not be suitable for your child's situation. The author assumes no responsibility for any adverse affects that arise because of the information presented in this book. The author has used the best efforts in assembling the information for this book, and makes no representations or warranties with respect to the information provided.

Bibliography

Batres, L. A. (2006). Beriberi. Retrieved from http://www.emedicine.com/ped/topic229.htm

Beach, C. B. (2005). Hypocalcemia. Retrieved from http://www.emedicine.com/emerg/topic271.htm

Beling, Stephanie. (1997) *Power Foods*. HarperCollins Publishers: New York.

Burger King Nutrition. (2006) Retrieved from http://www.bk.com/Nutrition/PDFs/brochure.pdf

Center of Disease Control (2006). *Physical activity for everyone: The importance of physical activity: Why should I be active?* Retrieved from http://www.cdc.gov/nccdphp/dnpa/physical/importance/why.htm

Dietary Reference Intakes (DRIs): Recommended Intakes for Individuals, Elements. *Food and Nutrition Board, Institute of Medicine, National Academies.* Retrieved from: www.iom.edu

Dietary Reference Intakes (DRIs): Recommended Intakes for Individuals, Vitamins. *Food and Nutrition Board, Institute of Medicine, National Academies.* www.iom.edu

Environmental Protection Agency. *What you need to know about Mercury in Fish and Shellfish.* Retrieved from www.epa.gov

Food and Nutrition Information Center (2006). Dietary reference intakes and recommended daily allowances. Retrieved from http://www.nal.usda.gov/fnic/etext/000105.html

Frye, R. E. & Jabbour, S. A. (2002). Pyridoxine deficiency. Retrieved from http://www.emedicine.com/med/topic1977.htm

Garth, D. (2006). Hyperkalemia. Retrieved from http://www.emedicine.com/EMERG/topic261.htm

Hemphill, R. R. (2006). Hypercalcemia. Retrieved from http://www.emedicine.com/EMERG/topic260.htm

Henry, C. L. & Schlach, D. S. (2005). Vitamin E toxicity. Retrieved from http://www.emedicine.com/med/topic2384.htm

Kleinman, R.E., Hall, S., Green, H., Korzic-Ramirez, D. (2002). Diet, breakfast, and academic performance in children. *Annals of Nutrition and Metabolism* (46) p. 24

McDonald's USA Nutritional Information. (2006) Retrieved from http://www.mcdonalds.com/usa/eat/nutrition_info.html

Novello, N. (2005). Hypermagnasemia. Retrieved from http://www.emedicine. com/EMERG/topic262.htm

Novello, N. (2005). Hypomagnasemia. Retrieved from http://www.emedicine. com/EMERG/topic274.htm

Patel, P. & Mikhail, M. (2004). Vitamin K deficiency. Retrieved from http:// www.emedicine.com/MED/topic2385.htm

Rosenbloom, M. (2005). Toxicity, vitamin. Retrieved from http://www. emedicine.com/emerg/topic638.htm

Rothschild, B. M. & Sebes, J. I. (2003). Scurvy. Retrieved from http://www. emedicine.com/radio/topic628.htm

Sloan, H. R. (2005). Biotin deficiency. Retrieved from http://www.emedicine. com/ped/topic238.htm

Strong, W.B, Malina, R.M., Blimkie, C.J., Daniels, S.R., Dishman, R.K., Gutin, B., Hergenroeder, A.C., Must, A., Nixon, P.A., Pivarnik, J.M., Rowlad, T., Trost, S., & Trudeau, F. (2005). *Evidence based physical activity for school-age youth.* Journal of Pediatrics 146(6) pp. 732-7

Tsiouris, N. & Ziel, F. H. (2002). Riboflavin deficiency. Retrieved from http:// www.emedicine.com/med/topic2031.htm

United States Department of Agriculture. How much do Americans pay for fruits and vegetables/AIB-790. Economic Research Service. www.ers.usda. gov/publications/aib790/aib790f.pdf

United States Department of Agriculture: Food and Nutrition Information Center, *Dietary Reference Intakes and Recommended Daily Allowances.* Retrieved from http://www.nal.usda.gov/fnic/etext/000105.html

United States Department of Agriculture. Cook it! *Food safety facts: United States Department of Agriculture food safety and inspection services. Retrieved from http://www.foodsafety.gov/~fsg/fs-cook.html*

United States Department of Agriculture. *My Pyramid.* Retrieved from www. mypyramid.gov

United States Department of Agriculture. *Official USDA food plans: Cost of healthy food at home at four levels, U.S. average, January 2007.* Retrieved from: http://www.cnpp.usda.gov/Publications/FoodPlans/2007/ CostofFoodJan07.pdf

Vohra, M., Gentili, A., Subir, V., Chen, D., Mosalem, A., & Siddiqi, W. (2004). Folic acid deficiency. Retrieved from http://www.emedicine.com/med/ topic802.htm

978-0-595-44939-2
0-595-44939-5

Printed in the United States
117129LV00010B/151/A